Sunnah Health

Embrace Prophetic Habits for Nutrition and Fitness to Boost Your Energy and Wellbeing

SARAH GULFRAZ

Copyright © 2025 Sarah Gulfraz

Sarah Gulfraz has asserted her right to be identified as the author of this Work in accordance with the Copyright, Designs and Patents Act 1988.

All rights reserved.

No portion of this book may be reproduced in any form, stored in a retrieval system, stored in a database, or published/transmitted in any form or by any means, electronic, mechanical, photocopying, recording or otherwise, without prior written permission of the publisher.

Dedication

~ Bismillah ~

May Allah (swt) accept our efforts and grant us success in this life and the next. Ameen.

In dedication to my loving family and all their support.

Contents

1. Introduction — 1
2. Introduction to Sunnah Nutrition and Fitness — 3
3. The Concept of Holistic Health in Islam — 21
4. Prophetic Dietary Guidelines — 29
5. Sunnah Superfoods and Nutritional Benefits — 40
6. Fasting (Sawm) and its Health Benefits — 52
7. Fitness and Physical Activity in Islam — 67
8. Spiritual Fitness and Mental Well-being — 77
9. Sleep Hygiene According to Sunnah — 93
10. Hydration and Sunnah Drinking Habits — 103
11. Implementing Sunnah Nutrition and Fitness Principles — 113
12. Conclusion — 125

Find Out More — 128

Chapter One

Introduction

In a world filled with conflicting information about health and wellness, it's easy to feel overwhelmed by the vast number of dietary trends and fitness programs. Yet, centuries ago, the Prophet Muhammad (PBUH) offered simple, timeless guidance on how to live a balanced and healthy life.

The notion of well-being in Islam encompasses more than just physical health. It includes our spiritual, emotional, and mental facets of being. This book takes a comprehensive approach to health and wellness, exploring Islamic principles that can empower us to strike this balance despite our hectic schedules. Offering practical advice for all Muslims – male or female, young or old – it serves as a guide to nurturing every area of our lives in alignment with timeless Islamic teachings.

We're extremely fortunate to have a religion that teaches us a comprehensive way of living. The Quran and the Prophet's (PBUH) Sunnah provide us with exquisite guidance on everything from marital relations to what to eat and how to behave during times of conflict. Mental well-being is considered an amanah (trust) from Allah (SWT). Since mental health affects how we think, feel, and act and how we manage stress, interact with people, and make decisions, it is our collective duty to learn more about how to have better brains.

As a result, many verses of the Quran and hadith (narrations of the Prophet's words, deeds, and character) deal with mental health and wellness and offer timeless guidance and advice that we can and ought to use in our day-to-day lives. This book aims to bring those prophetic teachings to the forefront, merging traditional wisdom with modern insights.

The Sunnah, the practices of the Prophet Muhammad (PBUH), encompasses various aspects of life, including nutrition, physical activity, mental health, and overall well-being. This eBook explores these practices in depth, highlighting how they can be integrated into our daily lives to achieve a holistic approach to health. Whether you're looking to improve your diet, enhance your physical fitness, or find spiritual peace, the Sunnah offers valuable principles that can help guide you on your journey.

From exploring prophetic dietary guidelines and superfoods to understanding the benefits of fasting and physical activity, this eBook will provide practical insights and tips to help you embrace a Sunnah-based lifestyle. By aligning our habits with the teachings of the Prophet (PBUH), we can cultivate better health, vitality, and a stronger connection with our Creator.

Let's begin this journey towards embracing the prophetic habits that can help us achieve optimal health and well-being in both body and soul. Ready to dive in?

Chapter Two

Introduction to Sunnah Nutrition and Fitness

Understanding Sunnah-Based Lifestyle Choices

Everyone has a unique way of living. Some individuals make intentional lifestyle choices in their fashion, diet, and activities. These preferences can be influenced by factors such as access, financial resources, or environmental conditions. Nonetheless, many lifestyle choices mirror a person's values and character, regardless of socioeconomic status, ethnicity, or environment.

For Muslims, living in accordance with their obligations to Allah (SWT) shapes their lifestyle, with the Five Pillars of Islam serving as core principles. Their lifestyle decisions are guided by Islamic teachings, aiming to follow Allah's (SWT) commands, find personal fulfilment, and contribute positively to society.

A Muslim's lifestyle is ideally rooted in the Quran and the authentic traditions of the Prophet Muhammad (PBUH). Islamic principles take precedence over national customs or local traditions in everyday practice. Much of the Muslim lifestyle draws from the Sunnah, the way of life exemplified by the Prophet Muhammad (PBUH).

In Islam, "Sunnah" refers to the practices, actions, and teachings of the Prophet Muhammad (PBUH), encompassing all aspects of his life and serving as a model for Muslims. It provides practical guidance on how to live in accordance with Islamic values and complements the Quran by demonstrating the application of its principles. The Prophet's (PBUH) Sunnah has been preserved through the Hadith—records of his sayings, actions, and teachings meticulously compiled in authentic Hadith collections.

> *The Prophet Muhammad (PBUH) is explicitly mentioned by Allah (SWT) as the best example for Quranic believers: There is indeed a good model for you in the Messenger of Allah (PBUH) for the one who has hope in Allah (SWT) and the Last Day, and remembers Allah (SWT) profusely (Quran 33:21)*

Like other daily issues, the laws around eating and drinking have been thoroughly covered in the Quran and the Sunnah, offering a comprehensive set of instructions that are both palatable to Allah (SWT) and good for one's health. The benefits of specific meals have been highlighted for optimal sustenance, and Allah (SWT), in His Infinite Wisdom, has made food essential for the survival and feeding of both mind and body.

Overview of Sunnah Practices Related to Nutrition and Fitness

Islam places significant emphasis on leading a healthy lifestyle, as physical and mental well-being are essential for inner peace and thoughtful living. Islam encourages the use of intellect in every area of life, recognising that clear thinking is only possible with a healthy mind. Therefore, maintaining both emotional and physical fitness is crucial for a fulfilling life.

Caring for our health and bodies is also a form of gratitude and responsibility, as we're all creations of Allah (SWT) and will eventually return to Him. Our bodies are gifts entrusted to us by Allah (SWT), and it's our duty to care for them responsibly. We're expected to return them in the best condition possible, avoiding neglect or harm. Respecting and honouring our bodies also aligns with the values of Islam and reflects our appreciation for this blessing.

> *Allah (SWT) says in the Quran: "O Children of Adam! Dress properly whenever you are at worship. Eat and drink, but do not waste. Surely He does not like the wasteful." (Quran 7:31)*

Numerous passages in the Quran offer guidance on eating well and the connection between spiritual and physical well-being. Warnings to remember Allah (SWT) and stay away from Satan are frequently coupled with encouragement to eat only excellent and pure food. Eating a healthy diet affects our ability to worship and satisfy our appetite.

> *"O mankind, eat of that which is lawful and good on the earth and do not follow the footsteps of Satan. Indeed, he is to you a clear enemy." (Quran 2:168)*

A person may become physically weak or lose focus on their main goal of serving Allah (SWT) if they develop a food obsession or overindulge in unhealthy or junk food. However, if one focused solely on spiritual pursuits and neglected their diet and physical well-being, they would also be unable to perform their required acts of worship due to weakness, disease, or injury. The teachings of the Prophet Muhammad (PBUH) and the Quran counsel humanity to balance these two extremes.

Eating Less – The Solution To Many Problems

> *Abu Juhayfah said: "A man burped in the presence of the Messenger of Allah (PBUH), and he said: "Keep your burps away from us, for the one who eats his fill the most in this world will be hungry for the longest time on the Day of Resurrection." (Al-Tabaraani–Saheeh)*

Abu Juhayfah (RA) practised remarkable self-restraint, abstaining from filling his stomach for thirty years; if he had breakfast, he would skip dinner, and if he had dinner, he would forego breakfast. In contrast, today, we often pressure our children—and ourselves—to eat until fully satisfied, not recognising the implications. Not only does overeating negatively impact health, but it also goes against the wise guidance of our beloved Prophet (PBUH).

Excessive eating leads to a sluggish body, promoting yawning and a lack of motivation, which can hinder our focus and devotion to worship. Moderation in eating supports both physical well-being and the clarity needed for sincere worship, helping us avoid distractions and laziness in our duties to Allah (SWT).

> *The Prophet (PBUH) said, "A believer eats in one intestine, and a kafir (unbeliever) or a hypocrite eats in seven intestines." (Bukhaari)*

> *The Prophet (PBUH) also said: "The son of Adam does not fill any vessel worse than his stomach. It is sufficient for the son of Adam to eat a few morsels to keep him alive if he must fill it, then one-third for his food, one-third for his drink, and one-third for air." (Tirmidhi)*

Not getting too comfortable whilst eating

The Prophet (PBUH) said: "I do not eat whilst I am reclining." (Bukhaari)

One reason often mentioned is that when we're very comfortable, we tend to overeat. In fact, some brothers in the Ummah today even loosen their belts to continue eating, which goes against the Sunnah's teachings.

Sitting in a position where the stomach is slightly compressed can help us feel full sooner, leaving part of the stomach empty, as recommended.

Unfortunately, there are generally two types of individuals. The first group, often the majority, consists of men who stay in shape and maintain fitness until marriage. After marriage, however, it seems they believe it's acceptable to let themselves go and become complacent.

We should strive to stay fit to be able to serve the Ummah whenever necessary. The second group is highly focused on their appearance and physique, sometimes prioritising their workout routine over other responsibilities, even neglecting Fard prayers at the Masjid.

True believers need healthy bodies and minds to worship Allah (SWT) properly. To keep a sound mind, a pure heart, and a healthy body, it's essential to prioritise health.

The heart and mind are nourished through remembrance of Allah (SWT), and worship is conducted in a lawful manner, while the body is sustained by consuming the pure, lawful food provided by Allah (SWT). Attention to diet and nutrition is an integral part of the holistic health approach embedded in Islam.

Sports for Strength

Engaging in permissible sports is highly beneficial for a believer, as it promotes physical strength and preserves health, which, in turn, supports one's ability to worship and strive for Allah's (SWT) sake. There are important Islamic guidelines to keep in mind when participating in sports and physical activities aimed at building strength:

- Seek Allah's (SWT) reward by engaging in these activities with the intention of enhancing your ability to worship Him and assist those who are oppressed.

- Avoid anything in sports that goes against Islamic principles, such as bowing to others, striking the face, uncovering the 'awrah, gambling, and other prohibited acts.

- Ensure that sports and exercise do not interfere with acts of obedience to Allah (SWT), respect for parents, and other essential responsibilities.

- Avoid excessive spending on sports; instead, practice moderation, keeping within the boundaries of Islamic teachings.

The Prophet Muhammad (PBUH) participated in physical activities such as wrestling with Rukaanah (RA) before embracing Islam. Abu Dawood narrated that Rukaanah wrestled with the Prophet (PBUH), and the Prophet (PBUH) was able to pin him to the ground (authenticated by al-Albaani in al-Irwaa).

Importance of Adopting Prophetic Traditions for Holistic Well-Being

Many refer to the dietary habits of Prophet Muhammad (PBUH) as the "prophetic diet" or "Sunnah diet." Rooted in Islamic tradition, this approach reflects his guidance on food and eating practices. Emphasising moderation, balance, and simplicity, the prophetic diet offers timeless principles for healthy living. While the concepts are broad, and interpretations may differ slightly depending on the source, its core components remain consistent. Here are some essential elements of the prophetic diet:

Moderation: The Prophet Muhammad (PBUH) stressed the importance of moderation in all areas of life, including dietary habits. He recommended avoiding overeating and filling the stomach entirely, as this could contribute to health problems and impact one's spiritual well-being.

To demonstrate this approach, the Prophet (PBUH) practised the habit of eating in thirds, refraining from excess. Similarly, the Quran cautions against indulgence in food and drink, encouraging a balanced, mindful attitude toward consumption.

Balanced diet: The Prophet Muhammad (PBUH) advocated for a balanced diet that included a variety of foods from different food groups. He highlighted the value of consuming fruits, vegetables, grains, and lean meats in moderation.

In addition to meat, the Prophet's meals included a range of other foods, such as dates, figs, grapes, milk, honey, olive oil, vinegar, watermelon, barley, pumpkin, squash, and various other available vegetables.

> *This is illustrated in a hadith, where Anas narrated: "A tailor invited the Messenger of Allah (PBUH) to a meal he had prepared. I went along with the Messenger of Allah (PBUH) where barley bread and soup containing pumpkin and dried sliced meat were served. I saw the Messenger of Allah (PBUH) reaching for the pumpkin around the dish, and since then, I have always liked pumpkins." (Abu Dawud 3782)*

This example underscores the significance of a balanced diet that includes a wide array of fruits, vegetables, and natural foods.

Certain foods hold a special place in Islamic tradition, as they were either favoured by the Prophet Muhammad (PBUH) or recommended for their benefits. For instance, dates and water are highlighted in numerous Hadiths (sayings of the Prophet) as nutritious choices. The Prophet also promoted the consumption of olive oil, honey, barley, and milk.

> *The Quran refers to the purity and value of milk, saying, "We give you drink from what is in their bellies - between excretion and blood - pure milk, palatable to drinkers." (Quran 16:66)*

Simplicity: The Prophet (PBUH) preferred simple meals over complex ones and was not picky about the type of food he consumed. Simple, healthy, natural items make up his diet. The Prophet favoured easily accessible and locally sourced foods.

Additionally, it's stated in the Quran that Allah (SWT) gives us food in the form of pure milk. It's said to be appetising to drinkers and is made from the guts of animals. This passage in the Quran emphasises how important it is to eat healthful, pure foods that are good for our bodies. We can ensure we give ourselves the best possible nourishment by selecting natural and unprocessed meals.

Fasting: During the lifetime of Prophet Muhammad (PBUH), fasting was an important discipline. In addition to its spiritual advantages, fasting helps the body detox and encourages self-control and moderation in eating.

The Prophet Muhammad (PBUH) highlighted the healing benefits of certain treatments and natural substances. He taught that healing can be found in three primary methods: cupping, honey, and cauterisation.

Cupping, an ancient therapeutic practice, involves applying suction to the skin to enhance blood flow and promote recovery. Honey, valued for its wide-ranging health benefits, is recommended as a remedy for various health issues. Cauterisation, a medical technique that uses heat to treat wounds or remove tissue, is also noted as a potential healing method. These teachings encourage the use of natural treatments in addressing health concerns.

> *The Prophet (PBUH) stated, "Healing is in three things: cupping, a gulp of honey, or cauterisation." (Bukhari)*

> *He also said, "He who eats seven 'Ajwa dates every morning will not be affected by poison or magic on the day he eats them." (Bukhari)*

Hygiene: The Prophet stressed the need for cleanliness and hygiene, which includes handling and preparing food correctly. To prevent contamination, he suggested washing hands before and after meals and ensuring food is prepared and kept properly.

Although the prophetic diet offers recommendations for wholesome eating practices, it's crucial to remember that everyone has different nutritional requirements and preferences. In addition to considering their personal health requirements and cultural customs, believers frequently adhere to the dietary ideals of moderation, balance, and simplicity.

It's essential to recognise that while the Prophet's (PBUH) dietary guidance offers insights into healthy eating, individual nutritional needs and preferences can differ. Many believers aim to embody the principles of moderation, balance, and simplicity in their food choices while also considering their own health requirements and cultural customs.

By following the Prophet's (PBUH) example, we can work towards leading a more balanced and healthful life. The story of the tailor inviting the Prophet (PBUH) to a meal reminds us of the joy and appreciation that can come from even simple foods.

The Prophet's (PBUH) fondness for pumpkins after that meal teaches us to be thankful for the blessings of food and embrace various nutritious options. Adopting the eating practices of the Prophet (PBUH) can benefit our physical health and deepen our connection to our faith.

Integrating Sunnah Principles into Modern Living

Relevance of Sunnah nutrition and fitness in contemporary lifestyles

> *Our beloved Prophet (PBUH) said: "The strong believer is better and more beloved to Allah (SWT) than the weak believer, while there is good in both." (Muslim)*

The relevance of Sunnah nutrition and fitness in contemporary lifestyles cannot be overstated, especially as Muslims navigate the challenges of modern living.

Our beloved Prophet Muhammad (PBUH) emphasised the connection between faith and health, illustrating the importance of both physical well-being and spiritual strength.

> *One such hadith states: "The strong believer is better and more beloved to Allah (SWT) than the weak believer, while there is good in both." (Muslim)*

This statement underscores the significance of maintaining a healthy body as part of one's faith and personal development. It reminds us of our responsibility to nurture our spiritual and emotional well-being but also to care for our physical health.

In contemporary society, the demands of daily life often create a disconnect between individuals and their physical health. With the rise of sedentary lifestyles, poor dietary habits, and increasing stress levels, maintaining a healthy body has become more challenging than ever.

However, the Sunnah provides a timeless guide to help us overcome these challenges and adopt a balanced approach to nutrition, fitness, and overall well-being.

The first key aspect of Sunnah nutrition is moderation. The Prophet (PBUH) instructed his followers to avoid excess in both food and drink. In a world where overeating and unhealthy food choices are prevalent, this principle of moderation remains relevant.

The Prophet (PBUH) often ate simple, wholesome foods, emphasising the importance of eating in moderation. He (PBUH) also encouraged the consumption of natural, whole foods, such as fruits, vegetables, dates, honey, and olive oil. These foods, rich in essential nutrients, form the cornerstone of a balanced diet in Islam.

One notable practice from the Sunnah is the principle of eating to benefit the body rather than indulge it. The Prophet (PBUH) would eat in small portions, often leaving some food on his plate, demonstrating the importance of being satisfied with what is enough. This is in stark contrast to the modern habit of overeating and consuming foods that are high in unhealthy fats, sugars, and processed ingredients.

Adopting Sunnah's approach to nutrition, which emphasises simplicity, balance and the avoidance of excess, can significantly contribute to improved health in the contemporary world.

Another key aspect of Sunnah fitness is physical activity. While the Prophet (PBUH) lived in a different era, the importance of regular physical activity was still emphasised.

The Prophet (PBUH) practised several forms of physical exercise, including walking, horseback riding, archery, and swimming, which were beneficial for physical health and provided a means of preparing for defence and strengthening one's character. In today's world, where physical inactivity has become widespread, the Sunnah offers a holistic approach to fitness.

The Prophet (PBUH) also encouraged his followers to maintain physical strength to serve Allah (SWT), protect the community, and be self-reliant. This principle of using physical fitness for service is highly relevant in contemporary society, where maintaining good health enables individuals to better serve their families, communities, and ultimately their Creator.

The benefits of physical activity are well-documented in modern science, and incorporating exercise into our daily routines is essential for preventing various chronic diseases, improving mental health, and boosting overall energy levels. The Sunnah's emphasis on physical strength and fitness thus aligns perfectly with contemporary knowledge about the importance of staying active.

Another practice rooted in the Sunnah that can positively impact our health is regular water consumption. The Prophet (PBUH) often emphasised the significance of drinking water in moderation and avoiding excessive thirst. He (PBUH) advised one to drink in three sips and not consume water too quickly.

In today's fast-paced world, many people lack enough water throughout the day, leading to dehydration, fatigue, and other health issues. Muslims can improve their overall health and well-being by following the Prophet's guidance on hydration.

Fasting, as practised during Ramadan, is another Sunnah with significant health benefits. While fasting is a spiritual worship act, it promotes physical detoxification and can contribute to weight management, improved digestion, and mental clarity.

Modern research supports the benefits of intermittent fasting, which has become popular for improving metabolic health. The Sunnah's approach to fasting teaches discipline, self-control, and mindfulness about our food choices, all of which are essential for maintaining a healthy lifestyle in today's world.

Furthermore, the Sunnah places great importance on the mental and emotional aspects of health. The Prophet (PBUH) promoted a balanced lifestyle, emphasising the importance of rest, relaxation, and maintaining positive relationships. Stress management and emotional well-being are key to overall health, and in today's fast-paced and often stressful world, following the Sunnah's guidance on maintaining inner peace, engaging in acts of kindness, and fostering strong social bonds is crucial.

The Prophet (PBUH) also stressed the importance of sleep and recommended a healthy sleep routine for maintaining physical and mental health. In the modern world, where sleep deprivation is a growing concern, following Sunnah's teachings on rest can help restore balance and improve overall health.

The Sunnah offers a comprehensive and timeless guide to achieving physical, emotional, and spiritual well-being. By following the practices of moderation in nutrition, incorporating regular physical activity, staying hydrated, observing fasting, and maintaining mental and emotional balance, Muslims can navigate the challenges of contemporary lifestyles while honouring the gift of their bodies.

The Sunnah's teachings on health and fitness are a means of improving individual well-being and a way to fulfil our responsibility to Allah (SWT) and lead a balanced, purposeful life.

Benefits of aligning health practices with Islamic teachings

Aligning health practices with Islamic teachings offers numerous physical, emotional, and spiritual benefits. Islam places great emphasis on the concept of balance, moderation, and the preservation of health, viewing the body as a trust from Allah (SWT).

> *The Prophet Muhammad (PBUH) said: "Your body has a right over you" (Bukhari)*

This emphasises that Muslims are responsible for taking care of their health and maintaining their well-being as part of their worship. This understanding is crucial, especially in contemporary times when health issues are on the rise due to poor lifestyle choices, unhealthy eating habits, and lack of physical activity.

1. Physical Health and Prevention of Diseases

Islamic teachings on health emphasise the importance of taking care of the body to prevent illness and promote longevity. The Quran encourages healthy living through moderation in all aspects of life.

> *Allah (SWT) says in the Quran: "Eat and drink, but do not be excessive. Indeed, He likes not those who commit excess." (Quran 7:31)*

> *The Prophet (PBUH) elaborated on this, saying: "The son of Adam does not fill any vessel worse than his stomach. It is sufficient for the son of Adam to eat a few mouthfuls that will keep him upright. If he must eat*

> *more, then let him fill one-third of his stomach with food, one-third with drink, and one-third with air." (Tirmidhi)*

This guidance from the Prophet (PBUH) reflects a fundamental principle in Islam: that overeating and excess consumption are harmful to health.

In today's world, where processed foods, sugars, and unhealthy fats dominate many diets, the Sunnah's emphasis on moderation is particularly relevant. It helps prevent lifestyle diseases such as obesity, diabetes, and cardiovascular problems.

Following the Prophet's (PBUH) guidance on eating in moderation promotes better digestion, a healthier weight, and improved overall physical health.

2. Encouragement of Physical Activity

The Sunnah also stresses the importance of maintaining physical fitness. The Prophet Muhammad (PBUH) engaged in various physical activities such as walking, horseback riding, archery, and swimming, promoting an active lifestyle that strengthens the body and mind.

> *The Prophet (PBUH) is reported to have said: "A strong believer is better and more beloved to Allah (SWT) than a weak believer, while there is good in both." (Muslim)*

This hadith emphasises that physical strength, in addition to spiritual strength, is highly valued in Islam. Regular exercise is not only a means of maintaining a healthy body but also a way of increasing one's ability to serve Allah (SWT) and fulfil one's duties.

This teaching is more important than ever in the modern era, where sedentary lifestyles are increasingly common. Regular physical activity—whether through walking, exercise, or outdoor activities—can help prevent a range of diseases and improve mental health.

Moreover, physical fitness enhances energy levels, focus, and overall productivity, enabling a person to be more effective in all aspects of life, including worship and community service.

3. Balanced Approach to Mental and Emotional Health

In addition to the physical aspects, Islamic teachings also offer guidance on mental and emotional health. The Prophet (PBUH) emphasised the importance of inner peace and balance, which are essential for overall well-being.

> *He said: "There is no disease that Allah (SWT) has created, except that He also has created its treatment." (Bukhari)*

This hadith reflects the Islamic understanding that all aspects of health—physical, mental, and emotional—are interconnected, and Allah (SWT) has provided remedies for them.

Islam encourages practices that promote mental and emotional health, such as maintaining positive relationships, showing kindness, and practising gratitude.

> *In the Quran, Allah (SWT) says: "Indeed, with hardship comes ease." (Quran 94:6)*

This verse reminds us that difficulties are temporary and can be overcome with patience and reliance on Allah (SWT). Practising gratitude, regular prayer, and connecting with others are ways to alleviate stress, promote emotional well-being, and cultivate a positive mindset.

> *The Prophet (PBUH) also encouraged Muslims to engage in Dhikr (remembrance of Allah SWT) to calm the heart and mind: "Verily, in the remembrance of Allah (SWT), do hearts find rest" (Quran 13:28)*

In times of stress or anxiety, this practice can bring peace and tranquillity, fostering emotional resilience and improving mental health.

4. Spiritual Well-being and Obedience to Allah (SWT)

Maintaining good health aligns with the spiritual teachings of Islam. Allah (SWT) has given humans the body as an Amanah (trust), and Muslims are required to take care of it as part of their submission to His will.

> *As the Quran states: "And do not kill the soul which Allah (SWT) has forbidden, except by right" (Quran 17:33)*

This verse not only forbids harm to one but also highlights the sanctity of life and the importance of protecting the body from harm.

Caring for one's body is an act of worship, as it is done in obedience to Allah's (SWT) commandments. When Muslims follow the teachings of the Quran and Sunnah regarding health, they are fulfilling their religious duties and seeking the pleasure of Allah (SWT).

> *The Prophet (PBUH) said: "Whoever eats, drinks, or does anything in moderation does so in accordance with the Sunnah of the Prophet (PBUH) and fulfils his or her religious duty" (Ibn Majah)*

This indicates that proper nutrition and fitness are integral to one's devotion to Allah (SWT) and a way to seek spiritual reward.

5. Long-term Benefits of a Healthy Lifestyle

Finally, the benefits of aligning health practices with Islamic teachings extend beyond immediate physical health. By following the Sunnah's approach to nutrition, exercise, and mental well-being, Muslims are also investing in their long-term health.

The Prophet (PBUH) was keen on preserving his physical health to ensure he could fulfil his mission, and he taught his followers to do the same. The longevity of a healthy lifestyle, built on the principles of the Sunnah, ensures that individuals can serve their families, communities, and Allah (SWT) for many years.

In conclusion, aligning one's health practices with Islamic teachings offers numerous benefits. By embracing the principles of moderation, engaging in regular physical activity, caring for mental and emotional well-being, and fulfilling our duty to Allah (SWT) in preserving our bodies, Muslims can lead healthier, more balanced lives.

The Quran and Sunnah provide a comprehensive guide to well-being, offering practical advice that remains relevant in the modern world. By following these teachings, Muslims can enhance their physical, emotional, and spiritual health, ultimately drawing closer to Allah (SWT) and fulfilling their purpose in life.

Chapter Three

The Concept of Holistic Health in Islam

Quranic and Prophetic Perspective on Health and Well-being

Islam places equal emphasis on both promoting health and protecting it. Health promotion in Islam encompasses a wide range of practices to improve and safeguard human well-being, including personal hygiene, nutrition, respect for the body, and the institution of marriage.

Health protection, on the other hand, involves measures to prevent infectious diseases, reduce the risk of injury, and avoid harmful substances such as alcohol, drugs, and tobacco. It also stresses the responsibility of parents, the importance of a healthy environment, the preservation of agriculture, and the role of the community in ensuring public health and preventing the spread of infections.

Islam introduced many principles of modern health promotion and protection centuries before they were widely acknowledged in contemporary times. In fact, only in the 20th century did the world begin to fully understand the importance of health as a fundamental human right.

This shift in perspective led to the recognition that every person has an inherent right to health, which should be universally respected and upheld. However, despite various international declarations affirming these rights, certain aspects of health – especially the rights of the human body – remain inadequately addressed in practice.

The value of Islam in this context is immeasurable, as it offers comprehensive guidance on health that has long been ahead of its time. It is crucial to delve into these teachings to understand and apply the principles Islam provides.

Allah (SWT) and the Prophet Muhammad (PBUH) have given us clear instructions and tools to protect our health, the health of others, and our environment. As such, we should recognise the power of religion and use the wisdom contained in Islamic teachings to care for our health, as well as that of our families, communities, and society at large.

By following the guidance of Islam, Muslims can take proactive steps toward ensuring the health and well-being of individuals and society. This can help achieve a collective effort towards healthier living and a stronger, more resilient community.

Importance of maintaining physical, mental, and spiritual health

Allah (SWT) has entrusted us with our bodies, and it's our duty to honour this gift by maintaining our physical health. This responsibility includes adopting practices that promote well-being, such as maintaining a balanced diet, engaging in regular physical activity, and ensuring proper rest.

As conveyed in his hadith, the Prophet Muhammad (PBUH) reminded us to eat and drink in moderation: *"Eat and drink, but do not be excessive."* This guidance teaches us the importance of moderation, leaving room in our stomachs for comfort and proper digestion and preventing overindulgence.

However, physical health alone is insufficient for a truly healthy life. True well-being encompasses not only the body but also the mind. The Prophet (PBUH) emphasised that good health extends to both physical and mental aspects of life. A person who is mentally and physically healthy is more capable of contributing positively to society, fostering strong relationships, and promoting personal growth. Mental health is just as important as physical health, and neglecting it can hinder a person's ability to live a balanced and fulfilling life.

Good mental health encourages joy, optimism, and a positive outlook on life. It helps one develop qualities like understanding, patience, and empathy, which are essential for harmonious relationships.

> *The Prophet Muhammad (PBUH) stated, "A strong believer is better and dearer to Allah (SWT) than a weak believer, while there is good in both." (Sahih Muslim)*

This hadith underscores that maintaining one's physical health contributes to general well-being and strengthens our ability to serve Allah (SWT). A healthy body allows us to fulfil religious obligations more effectively and engage in daily tasks with energy and focus.

Moreover, the Quran and Sunnah frequently emphasise the importance of mental and emotional well-being. Building inner strength through practices like mindfulness and seeking refuge in Allah (SWT) during challenging times is integral to our faith. Allah (SWT) commands us to seek peace through trust in Him, reinforcing that spiritual health is essential for coping with life's trials and maintaining emotional balance.

In summary, to honour the trust Allah (SWT) has placed in us, we must nurture our physical, mental, and spiritual health. By adopting a balanced lifestyle that includes physical activity, mental well-being practices, and spiritual mindfulness, we improve our quality of life, grow closer to Allah (SWT), and fulfil our purpose in this world.

Integrating holistic health principles into daily routines

Holistic health examines the connections between your emotional, spiritual, and physical well-being. Adopting behaviours promoting each area is essential to leading a healthy and balanced life. This creates a well-rounded daily schedule that includes self-care, mindfulness, and wholesome routines.

A daily routine is a collection of customs and behaviours one consistently adheres to. It ensures that significant activities are accomplished effectively and efficiently and gives one's life shape and discipline.

A daily routine is crucial in Islam because it helps guarantee that Muslims carry out their duties and commitments under the religion. A Muslim's daily schedule should be organised according to the Quran and Hadith.

> *The Quran emphasises the importance of prayer and states that Muslims must pray five times a day at specific times (Quran 4:103)*

The Hadith also offers advice on everyday routines, including getting up early, keeping one clean, and staying healthy.

Prayer: The most significant part of a Muslim's daily schedule is prayer. Five daily prayers are mandatory for Muslims, helping them stay in touch with Allah (SWT) all day. Additionally, prayer contributes to a sense of calm and peace, which is necessary for keeping a good perspective on life.

Getting up early: In Islam, rising early is one of the most significant parts of a daily schedule; rising early encourages Muslims to begin their day with prayer and remembering Allah (SWT).

Prophet Muhammad (PBUH) emphasised the importance of waking up early and stated that "Allah (SWT) made the early hours blessed for my Ummah." (Sahih Muslim)

Rest and Sleep: Getting enough sleep and rest is essential to staying healthy. The Prophet Muhammad (PBUH) stressed the value of getting enough sleep and advised taking a quick nap (Qailulah) during the day. He also urged getting up early for the Fajr prayer and cautioned against staying up too late at night. These practices align with recent studies that emphasise the benefits of maintaining proper sleep habits.

Cleanliness and Hygiene: The Sunnah strongly emphasises cleanliness and personal hygiene. The Prophet Muhammad (PBUH) advocated regular showers, clean clothes, and maintaining personal hygiene. These behaviours are essential for avoiding disease and fostering well-being.

Keeping Your Health in Check: Islam also stresses the importance of staying healthy. The Prophet Muhammad (PBUH) stated that "A strong believer is better and more beloved to Allah (SWT) than a weak believer" (Sahih Muslim). Muslims are urged to maintain good physical and mental health, exercise, and consume a balanced diet.

Slowly Eat and Drink: Our brain starts sending signs of fullness around 20 minutes after eating. When overweight men and women decreased their regular eating pace, they consumed fewer calories. Prophet Muhammad (PBUH) personally practiced and strongly recommended slow eating and drinking to improve digestion.

Including Islamic principles in your regular workout regimen is not only feasible but can also improve your physical and spiritual well-being. You can maintain your religious beliefs while enjoying the health advantages of exercise by beginning with appreciation and intention, being consistent, adhering to the Sunnah, seeking social support, and participating in philanthropic endeavours.

Achieving Balance (Mizan) in Nutrition and Fitness

In the pursuit of a healthy life, both physically and spiritually, balance (mizan) is an essential concept within Islamic teachings. The Quran and Hadith emphasise moderation in all aspects of life, including nutrition and physical activity.

Achieving balance in these areas is beneficial for our bodies and crucial for our spiritual well-being. Islam teaches us that the key to maintaining harmony is avoiding excess and practising moderation, whether in food, drink, or exercise.

Moderation in Food: Avoiding Excess

The Quran clearly highlights the importance of moderation in our consumption. Allah (SWT) advises us to eat only what is necessary and not indulge in excessive eating or drinking.

Overindulgence leads to both physical harm and disconnection from spiritual practices, as it can cause lethargy, make one less mindful, and impair the ability to perform acts of worship.

> *He said: "The son of Adam does not fill any container worse than his stomach. It is sufficient for the son of Adam to eat a few mouthfuls to keep his back straight. But if he must (eat more), then let him fill one-third of his stomach with food, one-third with drink, and one-third with air." (Tirmidhi)*

This Hadith encourages us to eat in moderation, limiting our intake to only what is necessary to nourish the body. It stresses that filling our stomachs with food, drink, and air is detrimental to our physical health, spiritual focus, and productivity.

Moderation in Exercise: Avoiding Overexertion

While food is vital for nourishment, physical activity is crucial for maintaining a healthy and balanced life. Just as overeating harms the body, overexercising can have a detrimental effect on physical health and mental well-being. The Prophet Muhammad (PBUH) emphasised the importance of maintaining physical fitness but discouraged extremes. He encouraged his followers to engage in physical activities such as archery, horseback riding, and swimming.

This serves as a reminder that we must treat our bodies with care, recognising that overexertion can lead to fatigue, injury, and an inability to maintain focus on our religious and daily duties. Excessive exercise can also interfere with our spiritual obligations, draining our energy from performing acts of worship like Salah (prayer). Achieving a balance between fitness and spirituality requires careful attention to both physical and spiritual needs.

Interconnectedness of Physical and Spiritual Health

In Islam, physical health is intimately linked with spiritual health. A balanced diet and regular exercise enhance our ability to worship, serve others, and fulfil our daily obligations. Conversely, neglecting our bodies can lead to sluggishness and neglect of religious duties.

This verse is a reminder that neglecting our bodies—through poor diet or lack of physical activity—is akin to harming ourselves. The body is a trust (Amana) from Allah (SWT), and we're responsible for maintaining it in the best possible state to serve Allah (SWT) and carry out our duties.

The Prophet Muhammad (PBUH) similarly taught that health and wellness are part of our spiritual responsibilities.

> *He said: "There are two blessings which many people lose: health and free time." (Bukhari)*

This Hadith encourages us to recognise the value of good health and use it to benefit ourselves and those around us. Proper nutrition and fitness allow us to be active, engaged, and present, fulfilling our roles as worshippers and community members.

The Role of Intentions in Achieving Balance

In Islam, the intention (Niyyah) behind any action is paramount. The pursuit of health and fitness is no different. If our goal is to improve our physical well-being to better serve Allah (SWT)—whether through worship, helping others, or fulfilling our family obligations—our actions are rewarded.

> *The Prophet Muhammad (PBUH) said: "Actions are judged by intentions, and every person will be rewarded according to what he has intended." (Bukhari)*

When we try to achieve balance in our lives—nourishing our bodies with wholesome food, exercising moderately, and maintaining a strong connection to Allah (SWT)—we align our physical health with our spiritual goals. This makes our efforts an act of worship, elevating the rewards of physical and spiritual well-being.

Achieving balance in nutrition and fitness is an ongoing process that requires conscious effort, mindfulness, and intention. By adhering to the principles of moderation and avoiding excess, we honour Allah's (SWT) trust in us.

As we focus on nourishing our bodies, we also strengthen our spiritual well-being, enabling us to fulfil our roles as worshippers and responsible stewards of our health. In doing so, we align our actions with the teachings of the Quran and Hadith, ensuring that our efforts toward physical fitness become a means of spiritual growth.

Chapter Four

Prophetic Dietary Guidelines

Prophetic Diet and Nutrition Principles

Islamic teachings on diet and nutrition are deeply rooted in the guidance of the Prophet Muhammad (PBUH), who emphasised the importance of balance, moderation, and maintaining good health through proper food choices. The prophetic principles on diet offer valuable insights that align with modern nutritional science, emphasising a holistic approach to well-being that encompasses not only physical health but also spiritual and mental well-being.

One of the most important principles in Islamic nutrition is moderation. The Prophet Muhammad (PBUH) advised against overeating, emphasising that one should eat only to the point of satiety but not overindulgence.

> *"The son of Adam fills no vessel worse than his stomach. It is enough for him to eat a few mouthfuls to keep his back straight. If he must [eat more], then let him fill one-third with food, one-third with drink, and one-third with air."*

This advice encourages portion control and balance in one's diet, preventing the negative effects of overconsumption, which is a common cause of obesity and chronic diseases today.

Islam also promotes the consumption of wholesome, natural foods that benefit the body. The Prophet Muhammad (PBUH) favoured simple, unprocessed foods such as dates, barley, olives, honey, and milk. These foods are rich in nutrients and provide essential vitamins and minerals. Dates, in particular, are highly valued in Islam, as they provide energy, are easy to digest, and are rich in fibre, potassium, and antioxidants. Honey, another food recommended by the Prophet, is not only a natural sweetener but also has numerous medicinal properties, including antibacterial and anti-inflammatory effects.

The Prophet Muhammad (PBUH) also encouraged the consumption of a variety of foods to maintain a balanced diet. This includes eating a mix of fruits, vegetables, grains, and proteins to ensure that the body receives all the essential nutrients it needs. For instance, the consumption of milk is recommended in many Hadiths for its health benefits, while the inclusion of fruits like pomegranates, figs, and grapes is often highlighted. In fact, pomegranate is mentioned in the Quran as a fruit of paradise, symbolising both its spiritual and physical benefits.

Islamic dietary practices also emphasise the importance of hygiene and cleanliness in food preparation and consumption. The Prophet Muhammad (PBUH) instructed Muslims to wash their hands before and after eating, a practice now recognised for its role in preventing the spread of bacteria and viruses. He also advised eating with the right hand, reinforcing the concept of cleanliness and respect during meals.

Islamic teachings also stress the importance of fasting, particularly during Ramadan. Fasting is seen as a spiritual discipline and a way to detoxify the body and promote physical health. The Prophet Muhammad (PBUH) recommended breaking the fast with dates and water, emphasising the importance of hydration and consuming easily digestible food to restore energy.

The prophetic diet and nutrition principles in Islam promote balance, moderation, and the consumption of natural, nutritious foods. These teachings encourage individuals to adopt healthy eating habits that support both physical health and spiritual well-being.

The emphasis on hygiene, variety in food, and moderation provides a timeless framework for maintaining a healthy lifestyle. By following these principles, Muslims can improve their overall health while honouring the teachings of the Prophet Muhammad (PBUH).

The Significance and Health Benefits of Sunnah Foods

Carbohydrates, proteins, and fats are three essential components of our diet. These three often spark debates and differing opinions among nutritionists and dieticians. While some emphasise the benefits of one nutrient over another, others caution against its consumption. Conflicting advice can feel overwhelming, as it often leads to confusion about what to eat.

A balanced diet, however, should consist of nutrient-rich foods that support overall health, bolster the immune system, and provide the body with the necessary vitamins and minerals to combat illness and infections. In this context, the Sunnah diet, as prescribed in the teachings of Prophet Muhammad (PBUH), offers a wealth of health benefits.

This diet promotes physical wellness and nurtures mental clarity, emotional stability, and spiritual health. As believers, we trust that Allah (SWT), in His infinite wisdom, has chosen the most nourishing foods for the Prophet (PBUH)—foods that modern science also recognises for their healing properties. The foods mentioned in the Quran and Sunnah provide profound health benefits, some of which are outlined below.

Honey is renowned for its medicinal properties, and its benefits are repeatedly highlighted in the Hadiths of the Prophet (PBUH). With its rich antibacterial, antiviral, anti-inflammatory, and antioxidant qualities, honey is an effective remedy for various ailments, including sore throats, coughs, and digestive issues. It has also been proven to speed up the healing of wounds and enhance the immune system's response. Honey gained significant popularity during the COVID-19 pandemic as a natural immune booster.

> *The Prophet (PBUH) once said, "Healing is in three things: cupping, a gulp of honey, or cauterization." (Bukhari)*

Dates were a staple in the Arab diet and are frequently mentioned in the Hadiths. The Prophet (PBUH) not only ate dates but also encouraged others to consume them for their health benefits.

Rich in essential nutrients such as fibre, potassium, calcium, and iron, dates are low in fat and cholesterol-free. Their high fibre content supports digestive health, while their vitamins and minerals contribute to overall wellness.

Dates are also known for protecting against toxins and harmful substances. Dates, especially the Ajwa variety, are also believed to strengthen the heart and promote a healthy digestive system.

> *The Prophet (PBUH) said, "He who eats seven 'Ajwa dates every morning will not be affected by poison or magic on the day he eats them." (Bukhari)*

Figs are low in calories and packed with nutrients, making them beneficial for bone health and weight management. They are especially effective in treating stomach disorders and improving digestion. Studies also suggest that figs can inhibit the development of cancer cells, making them a valuable addition to the diet.

The Quran mentions figs in Surah At-Tin, where Allah (SWT) swears by this fruit: "I swear by the fig and the olive." (Quran 95:1)

This highlights the fig's significance not only as a source of nourishment but also as a symbol of natural healing.

Barley is a versatile and nutritious grain that offers numerous health benefits. It helps treat fever, coughs, sore throats, and digestive issues. Barley's high fibre content aids in regulating bowel movements and promoting gut health, while its ability to combat hot-temperament illnesses makes it an excellent food for those recovering from illness.

A hadith narrated by a companion of the Prophet (PBUH) reveals that the Messenger of Allah (PBUH) entered upon us, and with him was 'Ali bin Abu Talib, who had recently recovered from an illness.

"We had bunches of unripe dates hanging up, and the Prophet (PBUH) was eating from them. 'Ali reached out to eat some, and the Prophet (PBUH) said to 'Ali: 'Stop, O 'Ali! You have just recovered from an illness.' I made some greens and barley for the Prophet (PBUH), and the Prophet (PBUH) said to 'Ali: 'O 'Ali, eat some of this, for it is better for you.'" (Ibn Majah)

Milk is mentioned both in the Quran and Hadith for its numerous health benefits. Prophet (PBUH) was known to prefer milk for its ability to strengthen bones, improve vision, and aid in the healing of ulcers.

> *The Prophet (PBUH) also recited a special dua when drinking milk: "O Allah, bless it for us and give us more." (Tirmidhi)*

> *The Quran also praises milk: "Pure milk, easy and agreeable to swallow for those who drink." (Quran 16:66)*

Milk's rich calcium and vitamin content makes it a vital part of the diet for healthy bones and overall well-being.

Pumpkins were a favourite of the Prophet (PBUH) and have several health benefits, particularly in treating heart diseases and certain cancers. Pumpkins are rich in vitamins A and C, and their high fibre content supports digestion and weight management. The Prophet's (PBUH) fondness for pumpkin is evident in a hadith narrated by Anas RA:

A tailor invited the Messenger of Allah (PBUH) to a meal he had prepared.

> *Anas said: "I went along with the Messenger of Allah (PBUH), and he ate barley bread and soup containing pumpkin and dried sliced meat. I saw the Messenger of Allah (PBUH) going after the pumpkin around the dish, so I have always liked pumpkins since that day." (Abu Dawud)*

Olives and olive oil are frequently mentioned in the Sunnah as beneficial for skin, hair, and overall health. Olive oil, in particular, is lauded for its anti-inflammatory properties and its ability to improve digestive health.

> *The Quran refers to olives as "the blessed tree" in Surah An-Nur: "And a tree that grows out of Mount Sinai which produces oil and a condiment for those who eat. For olive oil is the supreme seasoning." (Quran 24:35) The Prophet (PBUH) also said, "Eat of its oil and use it (the olives), for indeed it is from a blessed tree." (Tirmidhi)*

Melons are another refreshing food that the Prophet (PBUH) enjoys, especially when eaten with fresh dates. This combination of cool and warm foods helps balance the body's temperature. Melons are rich in vitamins and minerals, including vitamin C, which strengthens the immune system, and potassium, which supports heart health. Their anti-cancer properties further enhance their value in a healthy diet.

> *The Prophet (PBUH) said: "The heat of the one [melon] is broken by the coolness of the other, and the coolness of the one by the heat of the other." (Abu Dawood)*

In conclusion, the Sunnah diet is not only a reflection of the wisdom of Allah SWT but also an embodiment of natural health practices that continue to be relevant today. By incorporating these foods into our diet, we align ourselves with a legacy of healing and nourishment that benefits both the body and soul.

Foods discouraged in Islam

In the Sunnah, certain foods and dietary practices are discouraged or even prohibited, as they may not align with Islamic principles of cleanliness, health, or moderation. These foods or practices are highlighted through the teachings and habits of Prophet Muhammad (PBUH). Some of the foods discouraged in the Sunnah include:

Pork: Pork is strictly prohibited in Islam as it's considered impure. The Quran explicitly forbids it in several verses e.g., Surah Al-Baqarah:

> *"He has only forbidden you dead meat, and blood, and the flesh of swine, and that on which has been invoked the name of other than Allah; that which has been killed by strangling, or by a violent blow, or by a headlong fall, or by being gored to death; that which has been (sacrificed) on the altars (of idols); (forbidden is also) the division (of meat) by chance arrows: that is impiety." (Quran 2:173)*

Dead meat (Carrion): Consuming the flesh of dead animals (that were not slaughtered according to Islamic law) is prohibited. This includes animals that die from disease or accidents.

Blood: Consuming blood or blood products is forbidden in Islam. The Quran prohibits this in Surah Al-Baqarah 2:173 and other verses.

Intoxicants (Alcohol): Alcohol and any intoxicating substances are prohibited. The Prophet Muhammad (PBUH) strongly advised against drinking alcohol, as it impairs judgment and leads to harmful behaviours.

Excessive consumption of spicy or hot foods: While there is no explicit prohibition, the excessive consumption of overly hot, spicy foods is discouraged, as it can cause harm to the body. The Prophet (PBUH) promoted moderation in all aspects of life, including diet.

Overeating: The Sunnah encourages moderation and warns against overeating. The Prophet (PBUH) advised filling one-third of the stomach with food, one-third with water, and keeping one-third empty. This promotes better health and digestion.

Improperly slaughtered meat (not Halal): Meat that is not slaughtered according to Islamic law (i.e., not Halal) is forbidden. This includes meat from animals that were not slaughtered correctly or did not meet the halal requirements.

Eating in excessive amounts of delicacies: Certain foods like excessive sweets or luxurious dishes are discouraged if consumed in excess, as they can lead to unhealthy habits or indulgences that detract from moderation in Islam.

Rotten or spoiled foods: Foods that have gone bad or are spoiled should be avoided, as consuming them is harmful and goes against the Islamic principle of cleanliness and maintaining health. The dietary guidelines in the Sunnah emphasise the importance of consuming pure and healthy food in moderation. These central tenets of Islam promote physical well-being and spiritual purity.

Eating Habits and Mealtime Etiquette

The Prophet Muhammad (PBUH) imparted valuable guidance on the etiquette of dining, emphasising respect for food and moderation in its consumption. One of the core practices he (PBUH) encouraged was beginning a meal by invoking the name of Allah and concluding it with praise. This serves as an expression of gratitude for the nourishment provided. Eating with the right hand is also important, regardless of whether one is left-handed.

In the spirit of respect, the Prophet (PBUH) taught us to take the nearest portion when sharing a meal from a common dish, showing consideration for others. He also discouraged the use of extravagant items like gold or silver vessels and plates, highlighting simplicity and humility.

Hygiene and purity: The Prophet (PBUH) stressed the importance of hygiene in all aspects of life, including eating and drinking. He prohibited breathing into vessels and drinking directly from shared containers. These practices promote both spiritual rewards and good health, as well as proper etiquette.

Moderation and contentment: The Prophet (PBUH) practised moderation in eating, teaching that the food of two could suffice for three and that of three for four. His approach was to eat to live, not to live to eat. He often shared his food with those in need, demonstrating the importance of contentment and generosity.

Respect for food: The Prophet (PBUH) displayed a deep respect for food, always sitting upright while eating and avoiding lounging or reclining. He also emphasised that when supper is served and the call to prayer is heard, the meal should be prioritised before joining the congregational prayer.

Avoiding food waste: The Prophet (PBUH) strictly discouraged food waste, teaching that even a single morsel should not be discarded. He practised licking his fingers after eating to ensure nothing was wasted, reminding himself to appreciate every blessing.

Avoiding criticism of food: Criticising food was considered a form of ingratitude. The Prophet (PBUH) led by example, refraining from criticising food or pointing out its flaws. He would eat what he liked and leave what he did not, teaching us to avoid speaking ill of food and focus on gratitude.

Drinking manners: When it came to drinking, the Prophet (PBUH) recommended drinking water in three gulps and always mentioning Allah's name before and after drinking. Drinking while standing was generally discouraged, and eating while standing was considered even worse unless absolutely necessary.

Preference for certain foods: The Prophet (PBUH) had personal food preferences, such as dates, gourd, halwa, and honey. His meals sometimes consisted solely of dates and water. However, he (PBUH) never imposed these preferences on others. He also disliked foods with strong odours, like garlic and onion, advising caution when consuming them, particularly before attending mosques or social gatherings.

In a world where food wastage is rampant and millions face hunger, these etiquettes help cultivate gratitude for our blessings. By following these principles, we not only honour the divine gift of sustenance but also nurture our spiritual and physical well-being. May we continue to approach food with reverence, mindfulness, and compassion for those less fortunate.

Practising mindfulness (Tadhakkur) and gratitude (Shukr) during meals

Mindful eating and expressing gratitude before a meal send a signal to your brain that food is about to be consumed, allowing your digestive system to prepare for efficient digestion, nutrient absorption, and proper waste elimination.

Engaging in mindful eating supports a healthy body weight by encouraging you to be fully present with your meals and attuned to your body's hunger and fullness signals. This awareness helps you avoid overeating and makes you more likely to choose nutrient-rich foods. Slowing down and savouring your food not only promotes mindful choices but also reduces stress, improving both digestion and metabolism. This allows your body to avoid storing unnecessary calories.

In addition to enhancing digestion and nutrient absorption, mindful eating helps reshape your relationship with food, turning it into a more thoughtful, meaningful practice. When you approach meals with gratitude, you transform a routine activity into a sacred ritual.

By embracing these practices, you nourish your body with purpose, and align yourself with the natural rhythms of life. Next time you sit down to eat, take a moment to pause, offer thanks, and allow your meal to nourish you on physical, mental, and spiritual levels.

Chapter Five

Sunnah Superfoods and Nutritional Benefits

Concept of Halal and Haram

According to the Holy Quran, the term "halal" implies "permitted," "allowed," "legal," or "lawful," while its opposite, haram, signifies what is prohibited, illegal, or unlawful. Islam clearly identifies certain actions and items as haram, while others are deemed as halal. As Muslims, we should make every effort to adhere to what is allowed (halal) and abstain from anything that is prohibited (haram).

In the Quran, Allah said what Muslims are not allowed to do: "O you who have believed, eat from the good things which We have provided for you and be grateful to Allah if it is [indeed] Him that you worship. He has only forbidden to you dead animals, blood, the flesh of swine, and that which has been dedicated to other than Allah. But whoever is forced [by necessity], neither desiring [it] nor transgressing [its limit], there is no sin upon him. Indeed, Allah is Forgiving and Merciful." (Quran, 2:172-173)

Unless specifically forbidden by the Quran or Hadith, all foods are generally regarded as halal in Islam. According to Islamic law (Shariah), halal foods are defined as those that are devoid of any ingredients that Muslims are not allowed to eat.

Processed, created, manufactured, or kept using tools, machinery, and equipment that have been cleaned per Islamic law. One hadith states that if a person eats something that is forbidden (haram), Allah (SWT) will not accept their supplication.

Causes of Dietary Restrictions

A combination of spiritual, ethical, and health reasons inform Islam's dietary restrictions, which are intended to support believers' well-being and encourage a moral way of living.

Moral and spiritual purity: For Muslims, a ban on Haram foods contributes to their moral and spiritual purity. Individuals show their commitment to obeying Allah's commands and abstaining from immoral behaviour by refraining from eating prohibited items.

Ethical animal care: The ethical care of animals is reflected in the avoidance of carnivorous animals and raptors. Islam forbids actions that cause needless suffering to animals and promotes compassion towards them.

Well-being and health: Intoxicants, pork, and blood are prohibited to address hygienic and health problems. While avoiding intoxicants protects mental clarity and well-being, eating pork can put your health in danger due to possible parasites and infections.

Maintaining identity and faith: Muslims can uphold their unique identity and engage in their faith on a daily basis by adhering to dietary regulations. The connection between believers and their religious principles is strengthened by these limitations.

Islamic dietary customs heavily rely on the differentiation between halal and haram foods, which reflects a complex fusion of morality, religious convictions, and health consciousness. For Muslims, making a decision to follow these dietary regulations is a personal expression of faith and devotion, reflecting their dedication to leading a life consistent with their values and beliefs.

Advantages of Choosing Halal Food

Emphasis on quality and freshness: Halal food places a strong emphasis on freshness and high quality. Selecting halal options means choosing food that is carefully sourced and handled to meet strict standards of cleanliness and safety. The halal dietary laws focus on using fresh, natural ingredients while avoiding harmful substances like alcohol and pork products. This commitment to quality ensures that the food is free from contaminants and additives, promoting better health and well-being.

Rich source of lean protein: Halal meat preparation follows specific ethical guidelines that prioritise the humane treatment of animals, which are typically raised in natural environments and fed a nutritious diet. As a result, halal meat, particularly poultry and beef, tends to be leaner and a great source of high-quality protein. Lean protein is vital for muscle growth, tissue repair, and overall health. Including halal meat in your diet offers a healthier protein source with lower fat content.

Healthier fat choices: Halal dietary guidelines emphasise limiting the intake of unhealthy fats, such as trans fats, which are known to have a negative impact on health. Instead, the guidelines promote the use of healthier fat options, like those found in olive oil, nuts, and fish. These fats are beneficial for heart health and provide essential nutrients for the body.

Inclusion of whole grains and fibre: Whole grains like oats, brown rice, and whole wheat are commonly included in halal diets, offering a steady source of energy and helping to regulate blood sugar levels. The fibre content in these grains is also essential for maintaining good digestive health, thereby reducing the risk of various digestive issues.

Minimal processing for better nutrition: Halal foods typically undergo less processing, which helps preserve the natural nutrients and integrity of the ingredients. Unlike highly processed foods filled with artificial additives and preservatives, halal foods maintain a simpler and more natural composition. This reduction in processed ingredients contributes to a healthier diet and better overall health outcomes.

Cultural variety and nutritional balance: Halal cuisine reflects a wide range of cultural traditions, bringing together a diverse selection of foods, flavours, and cooking styles. This variety allows for a balanced and nutritious diet, providing a wide range of nutrients and the opportunity to explore new dishes. By embracing halal dietary practices, individuals can enjoy delicious and nutritionally balanced meals while also experiencing the richness of different culinary traditions.

From its focus on quality and freshness to the emphasis on lean protein, healthy fats, and whole grains, halal food supports healthy eating principles valued by many. Adopting halal dietary practices can help individuals achieve their nutritional goals while enjoying a variety of flavorful and wholesome meals.

Incorporating Sunnah Superfoods into Daily Diet

Recipes and dietary tips for incorporating Sunnah foods into meals

Incorporating Sunnah foods into your meals can be a wonderful way to nourish your body while following the teachings of the Prophet Muhammad (PBUH). These foods are known for their health benefits and can be easily integrated into daily meals. Here are some recipes and dietary tips for incorporating Sunnah foods:

Dates and Milk Smoothie

As mentioned, dates (especially Medjool) are packed with nutrients and are among the most recommended Sunnah foods. Combine them with milk for a nutritious, energy-boosting smoothie.

Ingredients:

- 5-6 Medjool dates (pitted)
- 1 cup of milk (dairy or plant-based)
- 1 teaspoon of ground cinnamon (optional)
- 1 teaspoon of honey (optional)

Instructions:

1. Soak the dates in warm water for 10 minutes to soften.
2. Blend the dates with milk until smooth.
3. Add cinnamon and honey, and blend again.
4. Pour into a glass and enjoy as a healthy breakfast or snack.

Dietary Tip: Dates are a natural source of sugars, fibre, and antioxidants, making them an excellent energy boost. The Prophet Muhammad (PBUH) often consumed them as part of his breakfast or as an energy source after fasting.

Olive Oil Dressing for Salads

Olive oil is another key Sunnah food known for its heart-healthy fats and anti-inflammatory properties.

Ingredients:

- 1/4 cup extra virgin olive oil
- 2 tablespoons balsamic vinegar or lemon juice
- 1 teaspoon mustard (optional)
- Salt and pepper to taste
- Fresh herbs (parsley or basil) for garnish

Instructions:

1. In a small bowl, whisk together the olive oil, vinegar, mustard, salt, and pepper.
2. Drizzle over your favourite salad of mixed greens, cucumbers, tomatoes, and olives.
3. Garnish with fresh herbs for added flavour.

Dietary Tip: Olive oil is considered a blessing in Islam. It benefits the heart and skin and reduces inflammation. Use it as your primary cooking oil or salad dressing.

Barley Soup

Barley is a nutritious, whole grain that the Prophet (PBUH) commonly consumed. It is high in fibre and can help with digestion.

Ingredients:

- 1 cup barley (whole or pearl)
- 6 cups water or vegetable broth
- 1 onion, chopped
- 2 carrots, chopped
- 2 celery stalks, chopped
- 2 cloves garlic, minced
- 1 teaspoon cumin powder
- Salt and pepper to taste

Instructions:

1. Rinse the barley under cold water.
2. In a large pot, sauté the onion, carrots, celery, and garlic until softened.
3. Add the barley, cumin, and broth (or water) and bring to a boil.
4. Reduce the heat and simmer for about 45 minutes until the barley is tender.
5. Season with salt and pepper, and serve warm.

Dietary Tip: Barley was a staple food during the Prophet's time. It is a versatile grain used in soups, stews, and salads. It is also known for supporting digestive health.

Honey and Ginger Tea

Honey, particularly pure, unprocessed honey, is another Sunnah food with antibacterial and healing properties. Ginger adds an additional layer of digestive benefits.

Ingredients:

- 1 tablespoon raw honey
- 1-inch piece of fresh ginger, peeled and grated
- 1 cup hot water
- Juice of half a lemon (optional)

Instructions:

1. Boil the water and add the grated ginger.
2. Allow it to steep for a few minutes.
3. Strain the ginger and pour the hot water into a cup.
4. Add honey and lemon juice if desired, and stir until the honey is dissolved.

Dietary Tip: Honey has been used since the time of the Prophet Muhammad (PBUH) for its medicinal qualities. It is great for soothing the throat, aiding digestion, and boosting the immune system.

Lentil Stew with Olive Oil and Vinegar

Lentils are rich in protein and fiber and were a staple in the diet of the Prophet (PBUH). This simple stew can be enjoyed as a hearty meal.

Ingredients:

- 1 cup dried lentils (red or green)
- 6 cups water or vegetable broth
- 2 tablespoons olive oil
- 1 onion, chopped
- 2 tomatoes, chopped
- 1 teaspoon cumin powder
- 1 teaspoon turmeric
- 2 tablespoons apple cider vinegar

Instructions:

1. Rinse the lentils and set aside.
2. In a large pot, heat the olive oil and sauté the onion until golden. Add the chopped tomatoes, cumin, turmeric, salt, and pepper. Cook for 5 minutes.
3. Add the lentils and broth (or water) to the pot. Bring to a boil, then reduce to a simmer. Cook for about 30 minutes until the lentils are tender.
4. Add apple cider vinegar and salt and pepper to taste.

Dietary Tip: Lentils are rich in protein and fiber, making them an excellent plant-based option for protein. Combined with olive oil, they provide a balanced meal favoured by Islamic traditions.

Sunnah-Style Grilled Chicken with Black Seed

Black seed (Nigella sativa), also known as cumin seed or black cumin, is mentioned in Hadith as a cure for every disease except death.

Ingredients:

- 4 boneless chicken breasts or thighs
- 1 tablespoon olive oil
- 1 teaspoon black seed (Nigella sativa), ground
- 1 teaspoon cumin powder
- 1 teaspoon garlic powder
- Salt and pepper to taste
- Lemon wedges (for serving)

Instructions:

1. Preheat the grill to medium-high heat.
2. Mix olive oil, ground black seed, cumin, garlic powder, salt, and pepper in a bowl.
3. Coat the chicken breasts with the spice mixture.
4. Grill the chicken for 6-8 minutes on each side until cooked through.
5. Serve with lemon wedges for extra flavour.

Dietary Tip: Black seeds have numerous health benefits, including boosting the immune system and aiding digestion. They pair well with grilled meats and can be added to various dishes for flavour and health benefits.

Promoting health and well-being through natural and nutritious choices

Promoting health and well-being through natural and nutritious choices is essential to living a vibrant and sustainable life. In today's fast-paced world, where processed foods and artificial ingredients dominate our diets, focusing on the benefits of consuming whole, natural foods is crucial. These foods, rich in vitamins, minerals, and fibre, not only support our physical health but also contribute to our mental clarity and emotional well-being.

One of the key principles of a nutritious diet is consuming whole foods that are minimally processed. Fresh fruits and vegetables, lean proteins, whole grains, nuts, and seeds provide essential nutrients for the body to function optimally.

For instance, fruits like berries, apples, and oranges are packed with antioxidants that fight inflammation and support the immune system. Vegetables such as spinach, kale, and broccoli offer vital nutrients like iron, calcium, and vitamins A and C, which are essential for maintaining bone health, boosting immunity, and enhancing skin health.

Whole grains, such as quinoa, brown rice, and oats, are excellent sources of fibre. Fibre supports digestive health, regulates blood sugar levels, and helps maintain a healthy weight. It also helps prevent chronic conditions like heart disease, diabetes, and hypertension. By replacing refined grains, like white bread and pasta, with whole grains, individuals can significantly improve their overall health.

Incorporating healthy fats into the diet is another vital aspect of promoting well-being. Healthy fats in foods like avocado, olive oil, and fatty fish such as salmon are essential for maintaining brain function, reducing inflammation, and supporting heart health. These fats are also a great energy source, which is necessary for optimal physical performance. By choosing natural sources of fats, individuals can avoid the harmful effects of trans fats and excessive saturated fats found in processed foods.

Moreover, natural foods are rich in the micronutrients—vitamins and minerals—that our bodies need to thrive. For example, vitamin D, which is essential for bone health and immune function, can be obtained from natural food sources like fatty fish and egg yolks, as well as from sunlight. Magnesium, which supports muscle function and relaxation, can be found in foods like nuts, seeds, and leafy greens. Ensuring a variety of natural foods are in the diet ensures that all essential nutrients are consumed in adequate amounts.

In addition to the physical health benefits, consuming natural and nutritious foods can profoundly impact mental health. Studies have shown that a diet rich in whole foods is linked to improved mood, better cognitive function, and reduced symptoms of depression and anxiety. The nutrients in whole foods, such as omega-3 fatty acids, B vitamins, and antioxidants, help nourish the brain, promote healthy neurotransmitter function, and protect against oxidative stress.

Ultimately, promoting health and well-being through natural and nutritious choices is about fostering a lifestyle that prioritises self-care and sustainability. By choosing natural foods, individuals not only nourish their bodies but also support their mental clarity, energy levels, and overall happiness.

These choices empower them to take control of their health and create a foundation for long-term well-being. Embracing this approach leads to a more balanced and fulfilling life, where food serves as a tool for healing, energy, and vitality.

Chapter Six

Fasting (Sawm) and its Health Benefits

Spiritual and Physical Benefits of Fasting

In Arabic, fasting is referred to as sawm. During the month of Ramadan, Muslims who have reached puberty must fast from sunrise to sunset, refraining from food, liquids, sexual activity, and offensive speech and behaviour.

> *"It was in the month of Ramadan that the Quran was revealed as guidance for mankind, clear messages giving guidance and distinguishing between right and wrong. So, any one of you who is present that month should fast, and anyone who is ill or on a journey should make up for the lost days by fasting on other days later. God wants ease for you, not hardship. He wants you to complete the prescribed period and to glorify Him for having guided you so that you may be thankful." (Quran 2:185)*

The night that the holy Quran was first revealed to humanity, known as Laylat al-Qadr (the night of decree), falls within the ninth month of

Ramadan in the Islamic calendar. As a result, Ramadan is a significant time for humanity and calls for Muslims to show extra devotion.

The foregoing Quranic verse highlights the deeper goal of fasting: to attain Taqwa or God-consciousness. Taqwa means seeking to abide by the morals and tenets of the faith at all times while remaining mindful of God's presence. The significance of maintaining this deeper commitment to self-control throughout the year can be emphasised by fasting.

The Prophet is said to have highlighted this wider dedication to self-control beyond food and drink in the two hadiths that follow:

> *"He who does not give up uttering falsehoods and acting according to it, Allah has no need of his giving up food and drink." "Fasting is a shield, so when one of you is fasting, he should neither indulge in obscene language nor should he raise his voice in anger. If someone attacks him or insults him, let him say: I am fasting." (Sahih Bukhari)*

> *"A man who does not guard his tongue, his hearing, his sight, and his limbs from forbidden acts during his fasting has, indeed, not fasted at all." (Makarim al-Akhlaq" by Shaykh al-Tusi)*

Understanding the holistic benefits of fasting in Islam

Fasting during Ramadan is a fundamental aspect of Islam, forming one of its Five Pillars. It's mandatory for all adult Muslims, except those with valid exemptions, to fast. Beyond its spiritual significance, fasting during this sacred month brings numerous benefits, including:

Enhanced Awareness of God (Taqwa)

Fasting during Ramadan nurtures a deeper consciousness of Allah (SWT), known as Taqwa. By abstaining from food, drink, and other physical desires from dawn until sunset, Muslims become more mindful of their dependence on Allah (SWT) and strengthen their self-discipline. This heightened awareness encourages a more reflective and conscientious lifestyle. The Quran underscores the purpose of fasting as a means to achieve Taqwa:

> *"O you who believe, fasting is prescribed for you as it was prescribed for those before you, that you may become mindful of God." (Quran 2:183)*

Developing Self-Control

Ramadan fasting is a practice that helps Muslims cultivate self-discipline by refraining from satisfying basic needs and desires. This restraint extends beyond physical needs to encompass control over emotions, promoting patience, humility, and the ability to manage anger. A well-known Hadith illustrates this concept:

> *"The Prophet (PBUH) said: 'Fasting is a shield. If someone is fasting, they should avoid using offensive language or acting in anger. If someone provokes or insults them, they should simply say: I am fasting.'" (Sahih Muslim)*

Fostering Compassion and Empathy

Experiencing hunger and thirst during the fast serves as a powerful reminder of the hardships faced by less fortunate people. This shared experience encourages Muslims to feel greater compassion and engage in charitable acts, strengthening their sense of gratitude. The Prophet Muhammad (PBUH) highlighted the importance of generosity during Ramadan:

> *"The Messenger of Allah (PBUH) was the most generous of people, and his generosity increased even more during Ramadan when the Angel Jibril (Gabriel) met with him." (Sahih Bukhari)*

Spiritual Renewal and Growth

Fasting provides Muslims with an opportunity for spiritual reflection and growth. By focusing on prayer, supplication, and self-reflection, they aim to cleanse their hearts and deepen their faith. This period of devotion helps them draw closer to Allah.

> *The Quran emphasises the comfort found in the remembrance of Allah: "Indeed, in the remembrance of Allah do hearts find peace." (Quran 13:28)*

Strengthening Community Bonds

The collective observance of fasting during Ramadan also helps unify the Muslim community. Sharing the experience of fasting, breaking the fast together, and participating in group prayers enhance feelings of connection and unity. This shared observance fosters a greater sense of belonging and mutual support.

> *The Prophet Muhammad (PBUH) encouraged praying together during Ramadan: "Whoever prays during the nights of Ramadan with faith and seeking reward, all their past sins will be forgiven." (Sahih Bukhari)*

Fasting during Ramadan offers a range of spiritual benefits, including heightened God-consciousness, improved self-discipline, increased empathy, spiritual growth, and stronger community bonds. Through this practice, Muslims are able to deepen their connection with Allah (SWT), enhance their understanding of their faith, and strengthen their relationships with one another, fostering unity and compassion within the wider community.

In addition to its spiritual significance, fasting in Islam also offers several physical benefits. One of the key advantages is detoxification and cleansing. By providing a break for the digestive system, fasting allows the body to focus on removing toxins. As food intake decreases, the body taps into stored fat for energy, which results in the breakdown of fat reserves that hold toxins, leading to a detoxifying effect.

Fasting also promotes improved metabolic health. It helps regulate blood sugar levels, insulin sensitivity, and cholesterol levels. During fasting, insulin levels decrease, and insulin sensitivity improves, which can help prevent type 2 diabetes and metabolic syndrome. Additionally, reducing insulin and blood sugar levels contributes to enhanced fat burning.

Weight loss is another common benefit of fasting. By reducing overall calorie intake, fasting encourages the body to use stored fat for energy, aiding in the burning of excess fat. Due to its effectiveness, intermittent fasting, which mirrors the fasting observed in Islam, has become a popular weight-loss strategy.

Moreover, fasting is linked to improved cardiovascular health. It can help reduce bad cholesterol (LDL), triglycerides, and blood pressure—key factors for maintaining a healthy heart and preventing cardiovascular disease. The discipline of fasting also promotes mindful eating, which can lead to healthier lifestyle choices overall.

Fasting enhances brain function by stimulating the production of brain-derived neurotrophic factor (BDNF), a protein that supports brain health and cognitive function. It also triggers autophagy, the process by which the body eliminates damaged cells. This helps reduce the risk of neurodegenerative diseases such as Alzheimer's.

In addition to these benefits, fasting can boost the immune system. It reduces inflammation, aids in the regeneration of white blood cells, and promotes the removal of damaged cells. This repair process strengthens the body's defence system, helping to protect against illness.

Fasting also supports better digestive health. Fasting can help alleviate disorders like acid reflux, bloating, and indigestion by giving the digestive system a chance to rest. It allows the system to reset and rejuvenate, improving gut health in the process.

Hormonal balance is another area where fasting has a positive effect. It helps regulate hormones such as ghrelin (the hunger hormone) and leptin (the satiety hormone), leading to better appetite control and healthier eating habits. Regular fasting, whether during Ramadan or as a voluntary practice, helps the body maintain equilibrium in hunger signals.

Studies have also suggested that intermittent fasting, like fasting in Islam, may increase lifespan and slow the ageing process. The autophagy process not only repairs and regenerates cells but also contributes to a longer and healthier life.

Lastly, fasting has been shown to reduce inflammation, a key factor in many chronic diseases. By allowing the body time to heal and repair without constant food intake, fasting helps lower inflammation levels, contributing to better overall health.

In Islam, fasting serves as both a form of worship and a means of improving physical well-being. Its benefits align with modern scientific research on health, making it a holistic practice that nurtures both body and soul.

Impact of Intermittent Fasting on Metabolism and Overall Health

Intermittent fasting (IF) has gained widespread popularity as a dietary practice involving alternating fasting and eating periods. This method is not only a modern health trend but is also rooted in spiritual practices, including Islamic traditions. Both scientific evidence and teachings from the Quran and Hadith support the health benefits of IF on metabolism and overall well-being.

Metabolic Benefits of Intermittent Fasting

Intermittent fasting (IF) affects the body at a cellular and metabolic level, promoting several health benefits. One of the primary impacts is on insulin sensitivity. During fasting periods, insulin levels decrease, which facilitates fat burning. Lower insulin levels help the body use stored fat for energy, potentially aiding in weight loss. Studies show that IF can reduce insulin resistance, lower blood sugar levels, and reduce the risk of Type 2 diabetes.

Intermittent fasting also influences metabolic rate. Improving hormone function can increase the release of norepinephrine, which boosts metabolism. This heightened metabolic rate can lead to increased fat-burning and weight loss. Furthermore, IF induces autophagy, in which the body cleans out damaged cells and regenerates healthier ones, aiding disease prevention.

Overall Health Benefits

The benefits of intermittent fasting extend beyond metabolism. It has been associated with improved heart health. By reducing factors like blood pressure, cholesterol, and inflammatory markers, IF contributes to a lower risk of cardiovascular diseases. Additionally, IF has been shown to positively affect brain health by increasing the production of brain-derived neurotrophic factor (BDNF), which supports brain function and may protect against neurodegenerative diseases like Alzheimer's.

Spiritual Perspective on Fasting

The concept of fasting is deeply ingrained in Islamic teachings. Muslims fast during the holy month of Ramadan from dawn until sunset. This spiritual discipline offers both physical and mental health benefits. The Quran states:

> *"O you who have believed, decreed upon you is fasting as it was decreed upon those before you that you may become righteous." (Quran 2:183)*

This verse highlights fasting as a means of attaining righteousness and self-discipline, which aligns with the physiological benefits of IF, such as improved self-control and eating habits.

> *The Prophet Muhammad (PBUH) also emphasised the importance of moderation in eating. He said: "The son of Adam does not fill any vessel worse than his stomach. It is sufficient for the son of Adam to eat a few mouthfuls, to keep him going. If he must fill it, then one-third for food, one-third for drink, and one-third for air." (Sunan Ibn Majah 3349)*

This Hadith reflects the principles of intermittent fasting, promoting mindful eating and preventing overconsumption, which can lead to metabolic disorders. Intermittent fasting is more than just a dietary trend; it is a practice that aligns with spiritual traditions and offers substantial health benefits.

By enhancing metabolism, improving insulin sensitivity, and promoting cellular repair, IF contributes to better overall health. Additionally, the teachings of the Quran and Hadith underscore the value of fasting as a means of self-restraint and holistic well-being, providing a timeless approach to health and spirituality.

Sunnah Practices during Ramadan and Beyond

Before the month of Ramadan, the Prophet Muhammad had a practice of only beginning his fast if he had seen the new moon or received trustworthy testimony of its sighting.

Sunnah fasting practices and traditions

Fasting (Sawm) is one of the key acts of worship in Islam. While obligatory fasting during Ramadan is well known, there are also voluntary fasts known as Sunnah fasting, which were practised regularly by Prophet Muhammad (PBUH).

These fasts are not only acts of devotion but also carry spiritual, physical, and emotional benefits. The Prophet (PBUH) emphasised these fasts as a means to draw closer to Allah (SWT), develop self-discipline, and purify the soul. In this section, we'll explore some of the key Sunnah fasting practices and their significance.

Fasting on Mondays and Thursdays

One of the most consistent practices of Prophet Muhammad (PBUH) was fasting on Mondays and Thursdays. He emphasised the significance of these days, stating:

> *"Deeds are presented to Allah on Mondays and Thursdays, and I love that my deeds be presented while I am fasting." (Tirmidhi)*

Fasting on these specific days is recommended for several reasons. Firstly, it aligns with the Prophet's practice and is a way to follow his example. Additionally, fasting on these days allows for regular self-reflection and accountability, as Muslims believe their deeds are evaluated weekly. The Prophet (PBUH) was known for his gratitude and mindfulness, and fasting on these days is an opportunity to express humility and dedication to Allah.

Fasting the White Days (Ayyam al-Beedh)

The White Days, or Ayyam al-Beedh, refer to the 13th, 14th, and 15th days of each Islamic lunar month, named for the bright, full moon that appears during this period.

> *Prophet Muhammad (PBUH) highly recommended fasting on these days, saying: "If you fast three days of the month, then fast the 13th, 14th, and 15th." (Tirmidhi)*

Fasting on these days is equivalent to fasting the entire month, as every good deed is rewarded tenfold. This practice provides a consistent worship routine beyond Ramadan, fostering regular spiritual discipline and a deep connection with Allah.

Fasting on the Day of Arafah

The Day of Arafah, which falls on the 9th day of the Islamic month of Dhul-Hijjah, is one of the most significant days in the Islamic calendar. It is the day when pilgrims gather at Mount Arafah during the Hajj pilgrimage, seeking forgiveness and making supplications. Fasting on this day is highly recommended for those not performing Hajj.

> *The Prophet (PBUH) said: "Fasting on the Day of Arafah expiates the sins of the previous year and the coming year." (Sahih Muslim)*

Fasting on this day is a powerful means of seeking Allah's mercy and forgiveness. It serves as a way for Muslims to spiritually connect with other pilgrims and participate in the sacred atmosphere of Hajj, even if they are not physically present.

Fasting on the Day of Ashura (10th of Muharram)

The Day of Ashura, the 10th day of the Islamic month of Muharram, holds great historical and religious significance. It is the day Allah saved Prophet Musa (Moses) and the Children of Israel from Pharaoh. The Prophet Muhammad (PBUH) encouraged Muslims to fast on this day and to add an additional day, either the 9th or the 11th of Muharram, to differentiate from the Jewish tradition.

> *He said: "This fast is a compensation for the sins of the past year."(Sahih Muslim)*

Fasting on Ashura is a Sunnah practice that reflects gratitude towards Allah (SWT) for His blessings and mercy. It is a day of reflection and an opportunity to seek forgiveness for minor sins committed in the previous year.

Fasting on the Six Days of Shawwal

After the completion of Ramadan, Muslims are encouraged to fast an additional six days in the month of Shawwal.

> *The Prophet (PBUH) said: "Whoever fasts Ramadan and then follows it with six days of Shawwal, it is as if they fasted for a lifetime." (Sahih Muslim)*

This practice emphasises the importance of consistency in worship and highlights the idea that the rewards for fasting extend beyond the month of Ramadan. By fasting these six days, Muslims continue the spiritual momentum built during Ramadan and demonstrate their dedication to Allah's guidance.

Fasting During the Sacred Months

The Prophet Muhammad (PBUH) also observed voluntary fasting during the four sacred months: Dhul-Qa'dah, Dhul-Hijjah, Muharram, and Rajab. These months hold special significance in Islam, and increased acts of worship are encouraged. Although fasting during these months is not obligatory, it's a means of earning extra rewards and drawing closer to Allah.

Fasting on Alternate Days (Fasting of Prophet Dawood)

The Prophet (PBUH) spoke highly of Prophet Dawood's fast (David), which involves fasting every other day.

> *He said: "The most beloved fasting to Allah is the fasting of Dawood; he would fast one day and not the next." (Sahih al-Bukhari)*

While this fast requires a high level of commitment and self-discipline, it's considered the best form of voluntary fasting due to its balanced nature. It neither burdens the person nor leads to neglect of other responsibilities.

The Sunnah fasting practices of Prophet Muhammad (PBUH) offer a pathway for Muslims to increase their devotion, purify their hearts, and gain numerous rewards. By fasting on specific days such as Mondays, Thursdays, the White Days, the Day of Arafah, and the Day of Ashura, Muslims can follow the example of the Prophet and strengthen their relationship with Allah (SWT). These practices are not merely about abstaining from food and drink; they are acts of worship that cultivate a deeper connection with the Creator, encourage self-discipline, and serve as a reminder of the greater purpose in life.

Following these Sunnah practices helps Muslims emulate the life of the Prophet (PBUH), bringing barakah (blessing) into their lives and fostering a sense of gratitude, humility, and spiritual growth. Sunnah fasting reminds Muslims that every moment offers an opportunity for worship and an invitation to draw closer to Allah (SWT).

Maintaining Optimal Health and Hydration During Fasting Periods

During the month of Ramadan, all Muslims endure hunger and thirst for over 12 hours a day. As a result, the body needs enough water and vitamins. Furthermore, the requirement to increase worship and rise in the middle of the night for the pre-dawn meal (suhoor) can cause abnormal sleeping habits.

Fasting can have various positive health benefits, especially when approached with a balanced mindset. It has been shown to help reduce risk factors for heart disease, particularly among overweight individuals. This includes lowering blood pressure and reducing LDL, commonly referred to as "bad cholesterol." Additionally, fasting can aid in improving liver function, boosting metabolism, and enhancing digestion.

To fully reap these benefits, you must maintain good nutrition and hydration throughout fasting. By focusing on balanced meals during the pre-dawn (suhoor) and breaking fast (iftar), you can provide your body with the necessary energy and stamina to continue your daily activities, even while observing a fast.

Fasting can present challenges due to changes in eating and sleeping patterns, which differ from a regular daily routine. Aside from managing hunger and thirst for extended hours, maintaining good health during fasting is essential to avoid falling ill. Proper planning makes it possible to stay healthy and active throughout this period. Below are some strategies to help maintain your well-being while fasting.

1. Incorporate light exercise

Physical activity remains crucial for both physical and mental well-being, even during fasting. Engaging in light exercise, such as walking, cycling, or jogging for about 30 minutes daily, can help boost metabolism and maintain fitness levels. To stay hydrated and safe, it's important to schedule this exercise at optimal times, such as after breaking the fast or in the early evening. Avoid strenuous activities during the day when your body is more prone to dehydration.

2. Focus on balanced nutrition

Ensuring a balanced diet during fasting is key to maintaining your health. Prioritise the intake of fresh fruits, vegetables, and lean protein sources, whether plant-based or animal-based. Foods high in fibre, such as whole grains and legumes, can help sustain energy levels and prevent digestive issues like constipation. It's best to avoid heavy, fatty, or difficult-to-digest foods, as these can cause discomfort and make it harder to stay active throughout the day. Opt for light, nutritious meals that provide the body with essential nutrients without causing bloating or lethargy.

3. Stay hydrated

Hydration is critical during fasting, especially since you cannot drink water throughout the day. To prevent dehydration, drink plenty of water between iftar and suhoor. Aim for at least 8 cups of water during this time. Additionally, coconut water can be an excellent option to replenish lost electrolytes. Avoid beverages like soda, coffee, or sugary drinks, as they can lead to quicker dehydration and leave you feeling tired.

4. Get adequate rest

Maintaining a good sleep schedule during fasting can be challenging but crucial for your overall health. Aim to get sufficient rest between iftar and suhoor, as lack of sleep can weaken your immune system and leave you feeling fatigued. If possible, establish a consistent sleep pattern, going to bed and waking up at the same time each day. Avoid staying late, as this can lead to exhaustion, making it harder to maintain your energy levels throughout the day. Proper rest is vital for maintaining focus, especially during prayer and other worship activities.

5. Plan a balanced suhoor

The pre-dawn meal, or suhoor, is crucial in helping you sustain energy during the fasting hours. Ensure your suhoor includes a balanced mix of complex carbohydrates, proteins, healthy fats, and fibre. For instance, you might choose oatmeal topped with fresh fruit, boiled eggs, or whole wheat bread paired with cheese or nut butter. These foods provide a steady release of energy, keeping you full for longer and supporting your body's needs throughout the day.

These tips will help you maintain good health during fasting and make the most of this spiritually significant period. A well-rounded approach, including balanced meals, adequate hydration, sufficient rest, and gentle exercise, can help preserve your vitality and well-being.

Chapter Seven

Fitness and Physical Activity in Islam

Importance of Physical Fitness in Islamic Teachings

Islam places a high value on living a healthy life, recognising that good health is essential for inner peace.

Since Islam emphasises the importance of reflection in all facets of life, it acknowledges that a healing mind is crucial for sound judgment and decision-making. Thus, to live a better life, one needs to be both emotionally and physically fit.

As mentioned earlier on in this book, we should take care of our bodies and health because we're all part of Allah (SWT), to whom we should return, and because Allah (SWT) gave us our bodies, which we should one day offer to Him.

Therefore, it's our responsibility to care for the bodies given to us and to offer them to Allah (SWT) in better shape. Our bodies don't deserve to be mistreated.

Prophetic Encouragement for Maintaining Physical Strength and Agility

In Islam, maintaining physical strength and agility is highly encouraged, as it contributes to overall well-being and enables a believer to serve Allah (SWT) more effectively.

Here are some prophetic teachings and Islamic principles that provide encouragement for keeping the body strong and healthy:

> *The Prophet Muhammad (PBUH) reminded believers that the body is a trust (amanah) given by Allah, and it is our responsibility to care for it. In a hadith, the Prophet said: "Your body has a right over you." (Sahih Bukhari)*

This highlights the importance of maintaining good health, which includes regular exercise, proper nutrition, and sufficient rest. Keeping physically fit allows us to fulfil our spiritual and worldly duties more effectively.

The Prophet Muhammad (PBUH) emphasised the value of strength in a believer.

> *He said: "The strong believer is better and more beloved to Allah than the weak believer, while there is good in both." (Sahih Muslim)*

This hadith encourages Muslims to strive for physical strength and vitality. Strength is not only about physical power but also mental resilience and spiritual fortitude. Physical strength, in this context, aids in perseverance and endurance in worship, charity, and serving the community.

The Prophet (PBUH) and his companions engaged in various physical activities that promoted health and agility, such as horseback riding, archery, and swimming.

> *The Prophet said: "Teach your children swimming, archery, and horse riding." (Musnad Ahmad)*

These activities are examples of sports that build physical strength, coordination, and endurance. They also reflect the Prophet's encouragement for Muslims to be active and maintain their fitness.

Walking was a common practice of the Prophet Muhammad (PBUH). It is narrated that he would walk briskly and energetically, which demonstrates his physical fitness and agility. The Prophet's pace in walking was described as purposeful, reflecting his discipline and vigour. Walking is a simple yet effective way to maintain physical health and is encouraged as a part of everyday life.

Islam promotes balance and moderation in all aspects of life, including physical health. Over-exertion or negligence of one's health are both discouraged. The Prophet Muhammad (PBUH) set an example of moderation and self-care.

> *He advised: "Take up good deeds only as much as you are able, for the best deeds are those done regularly even if they are few." (Sahih Bukhari)*

This principle can also be applied to physical fitness; consistent, moderate exercise is more beneficial than sporadic, intense exertion.

The Prophet (PBUH) emphasised mindful eating, a key aspect of maintaining physical health.

> "The son of Adam does not fill any vessel worse than his stomach. It is sufficient for the son of Adam to eat a few mouthfuls to keep his spine straight. But if he must eat more, then a third for his food, a third for his drink, and a third for his breath." (Sunan Ibn Majah)

This hadith highlights the importance of moderation in eating, which directly impacts physical strength, agility, and overall health.

The daily prayers (Salah) are not only acts of worship but also involve physical movement that promotes flexibility and strength. Bowing, prostrating, and standing help improve circulation, posture, and muscle health. Regular prayer, therefore, is a means of maintaining both spiritual and physical well-being.

The Prophet Muhammad (PBUH) often made supplications for health and strength. One such dua is:

> "O Allah, grant my body health, O Allah, grant my hearing health, and grant my sight health." (Sunan Abu Dawood)

Seeking Allah's help (SWT) in maintaining physical strength and good health is an act of faith and reliance on Him.

Islam encourages a holistic approach to health that integrates physical, mental, and spiritual well-being. By maintaining physical strength and agility, a believer can better fulfil their responsibilities, engage in worship with vigour, and serve the community effectively. The teachings of the Prophet Muhammad (PBUH) remind us that a strong and healthy body is a gift from Allah that should be nurtured and cared for with gratitude. May Allah grant us the strength and health to serve Him best and use our physical abilities for good, Ameen.

Benefits of regular exercise for overall health and well-being

Regular exercise has immense benefits for both physical and mental well-being, which aligns with Islamic teachings, which emphasise the importance of maintaining a healthy body and mind. In Islam, the body is considered a trust (Amanah) from Allah, and taking care of it is seen as an act of worship. The Prophet Muhammad (PBUH) encouraged physical activity, understanding that a healthy body enables a person to perform their religious duties effectively and live a productive life.

The Quran indirectly speaks of the importance of physical health through verses highlighting the body's greatness and its role in a believer's life. In Surah Al-Baqarah, Allah reminds us that He does not burden a soul beyond what it can bear:

> *"Allah does not burden a soul beyond that it can bear."*
> *(Quran 2:286)*

This encourages us to maintain our health so that we can handle the challenges that life presents, both physically and spiritually.

The Prophet Muhammad (PBUH) also encouraged physical strength and well-being.

> *He said, "A strong believer is better and more beloved to Allah than a weak believer, while there is good in both."*
> *(Sahih Muslim)*

This hadith highlights the value of strength, not just in physical prowess but in the ability to serve Allah and carry out one's duties with vigour.

Regular exercise contributes significantly to overall physical health. It strengthens the muscles, boosts the immune system, and promotes cardiovascular health. The Prophet (PBUH) was known to engage in physical activities, such as horseback riding, archery, and swimming, which are examples of exercise that promote fitness and endurance. Engaging in such activities enhances strength and improves one's ability to perform acts of worship, such as prayer, which requires physical endurance, flexibility, and focus.

Exercise also plays a critical role in mental and emotional well-being. The Quran frequently emphasises the importance of maintaining a balanced and peaceful state of mind.

> *In Surah Ar-Ra'd, Allah says: "Those who have believed and whose hearts are assured by the remembrance of Allah. Indeed, by the remembrance of Allah, hearts are assured." (Quran 13:28)*

Regular physical activity, especially when paired with prayer and remembrance of Allah (Dhikr), promotes mental clarity, reduces stress, and fosters a sense of tranquillity and contentment. The physical benefits of exercise are thus interconnected with spiritual well-being.

Moreover, physical activity helps alleviate feelings of stress, anxiety, and depression. Exercising releases endorphins, which are known to improve mood and reduce anxiety. This aligns with the Islamic concept of maintaining a sound mind and heart.

The Prophet (PBUH) taught that seeking a balance between physical, mental, and spiritual health is essential for a fulfilling life. Islam does not view physical health in isolation but encourages a holistic approach to well-being that nurtures the body, mind, and soul.

Exercise also promotes longevity and vitality, enabling a person to serve their community and family with energy and enthusiasm. In Islam, there is a great emphasis on fulfilling one's responsibilities toward others. A physically healthy person is better able to care for others, whether it be family, friends, or the wider community.

Finally, regular exercise can be a way of thanking Allah for the gift of good health. In Surah Al-Mulk, Allah reminds us:

> *"It is He who has made the earth subservient to you, so traverse in its tracks and partake of the sustenance which He has provided." (Quran 67:15)*

By taking care of our bodies through regular exercise, we fulfil our duty as stewards of our health, showing gratitude to Allah for the strength He has granted us.

In sum, regular exercise is not just a physical necessity but an integral part of leading a balanced and fulfilling life in Islam. It enhances physical health, fosters mental well-being, and deepens spiritual strength, all contributing to a life of purpose, productivity, and gratitude.

Sunnah Exercises and Physical Activities

Physical fitness has always been an integral part of human well-being, and Islam, as a comprehensive way of life, encourages both spiritual and physical health. The Prophet Muhammad (PBUH) not only emphasised the importance of maintaining a strong body but also practised various physical activities that became part of his Sunnah.

These activities are not only beneficial for the body but also for the soul, as they serve as a means to strengthen discipline, patience, and connection with Allah. This article explores examples of physical activities practised by the Prophet Muhammad (PBUH) and how we can incorporate these Sunnah exercises into our modern fitness routines.

Physical Activities Practised by the Prophet (PBUH)

Walking: Walking was one of the most common forms of physical activity practised by the Prophet Muhammad (PBUH). He often walked to places such as the mosque and marketplace and enjoyed walking while on his travels. His walking style was described as brisk but balanced, neither too fast nor too slow. He used to walk with his head slightly lowered, which is said to improve posture and balance.

> *"The son of Adam has no better remedy than walking, and whoever walks in the path of Allah, Allah will make his path easy to Jannah." (Sahih Muslim)*

Running: The Prophet Muhammad (PBUH) was also known for his ability to run swiftly. On several occasions, he engaged in races with his wives and companions.

It is recorded that the Prophet (PBUH) participated in a race with his wife, Aisha (RA), after their marriage. This light-hearted competition shows the importance of maintaining an active lifestyle while nurturing healthy relationships.

Horseback riding: The Prophet Muhammad (PBUH) practised horseback riding and encouraged it as a means of strengthening one's physical health and preparing for battle.

> *"Teach your children swimming, archery, and horseback riding." (Sahih Muslim)*

Archery: Archery was another activity that the Prophet (PBUH) practised himself and encouraged his companions to learn. He recognised the importance of archery in building both physical and mental discipline.

> *"The strong man is not the one who can overpower others in wrestling, but the one who controls himself in a fit of rage." (Sahih Bukhari)*

Swimming: Swimming is another form of physical activity encouraged in Islam. While it's not mentioned explicitly in the Hadiths of the Prophet Muhammad (PBUH), scholars and Islamic teachers emphasise the importance of this full-body workout. Swimming promotes cardiovascular health, flexibility, and muscular endurance. The Prophet (PBUH) is believed to have encouraged swimming, an activity that early Muslims practised.

Incorporating Sunnah Exercises into Modern Fitness Routines

In today's fast-paced world, it's easy to forget the simple yet effective forms of exercise practised by the Prophet Muhammad (PBUH). However, many Sunnah activities can be seamlessly incorporated into modern fitness routines to promote physical health and spiritual well-being.

Walking: Walking is one of the easiest ways to incorporate a Sunnah exercise into modern life. Many people today live sedentary lifestyles due to desk jobs and limited physical activity. Walking can be a powerful tool for maintaining good health, whether for leisure or commuting.

Walking for 30 minutes daily can help reduce the risk of chronic diseases, improve circulation, and even lower stress levels. In addition, walking outdoors provides a chance to connect with nature and engage in mindfulness, aligning with the peaceful reflection emphasised in Islamic teachings.

Group running or cycling: Participating in group fitness activities such as marathons or charity walks can emulate the physical and social benefits the Prophet (PBUH) experienced through his physical competitions. These activities improve cardiovascular health, build endurance, and create opportunities for community engagement. The camaraderie from group physical activities also reflects the spirit of unity in Islam.

Engaging in archery: In modern times, archery has experienced a resurgence as a sport and a form of physical exercise. For those interested in practising archery, local clubs and organisations offer training that aligns with the discipline the Prophet Muhammad (PBUH) encouraged. Archery can improve focus, enhance upper body strength, and foster a sense of patience and resilience.

Similarly, engaging in sports requiring strategy and teamwork—such as soccer, basketball, or even martial arts—can help instil values of discipline, perseverance, and cooperation integral to Sunnah teachings.

Swimming as a full-body workout: Swimming is a low-impact exercise that engages nearly every muscle group. It's a great option for those who may have joint issues or prefer non-weight-bearing exercises. Incorporating swimming into a fitness routine helps to improve muscle strength, cardiovascular endurance, and mental focus—all qualities that align with the physical health encouraged in Islam.

The Sunnah provides a wealth of guidance on how physical fitness can be a part of everyday life. The Prophet Muhammad (PBUH) not only practised various physical activities but also promoted their benefits to his companions. By incorporating simple exercises such as walking, running, swimming, archery, and cycling into our modern fitness routines, we can honour Islam's teachings and promote a balanced, healthy lifestyle.

These activities are not just about physical health—they serve as reminders of the discipline, patience, and spiritual growth that come with maintaining a strong and healthy body.

Chapter Eight

Spiritual Fitness and Mental Well-being

Spirituality, in the context of Islam, is the deep connection and devotion one has to Allah (SWT) and the sense of purpose and meaning in life that stems from this relationship. The Quran and Hadith emphasise the importance of nurturing one's inner self and seeking closeness to Allah to find peace, tranquility, and fulfilment in life.

> *Allah (SWT) says in the Quran: "Indeed, in the remembrance of Allah do hearts find rest." (Al-Ra'd 13:28)*

This verse highlights how spirituality—through the remembrance of Allah—brings peace to the heart and mind. Connecting with the Creator and seeking meaning through worship and good deeds is central to mental and spiritual well-being.

> *The Prophet Muhammad (PBUH) said in a Hadith: "Whoever is focused on Allah, Allah will make a way for him from every distress and will grant him relief from every hardship." (Sunan Ibn Majah)*

This Hadith reflects the idea that spirituality, through sincere devotion and trust in Allah, can provide solace and relief from the struggles of life. It encourages the believer to seek strength and purpose through faith, whether or not they follow a particular religious tradition, as the essence of spirituality is a connection to Allah and the pursuit of His pleasure.

Spiritual and Physical Fitness

In Islam, the concept of maintaining both physical and spiritual well-being is deeply interconnected. The body is a trust from Allah (SWT), and taking care of it is a form of worship. Just as we nurture our spiritual health through prayer and remembrance of Allah, we're encouraged to care for our physical health through exercise. Exercise can become more than just a physical activity—it can serve as a form of meditation and prayer, helping to deepen our connection to Allah and enhance our overall well-being.

Focusing the mind and heart

Physical activity offers a powerful way to achieve focus and mindfulness. Whether walking, running, or practising yoga, exercise lets you clear your mind and focus on the present moment. This single-minded focus can parallel the concentration required in prayer (Salah) and Dhikr (remembrance of Allah). By dedicating your attention to the activity, you align your physical and mental state, creating a space for spiritual reflection.

> *The Prophet Muhammad (PBUH) said: "A strong believer is better and more beloved to Allah than a weak believer, while there is good in both." (Sahih Muslim)*

This hadith encourages believers to strive for spiritual and physical strength, as both are valuable to Allah.

Expressing gratitude for the gift of health

In Islam, gratitude (shukr) is a fundamental aspect of faith. Physical activity, such as exercise, is a means of showing gratitude for the health and vitality that Allah has granted.

Each step, each movement, can be seen as an act of worship when done with the intention of maintaining and strengthening the body that Allah has entrusted to you. Taking care of one's health is a way of acknowledging Allah's blessings and fulfilling the duty to safeguard the body.

> *"And [remember] when your Lord proclaimed: 'If you give thanks [by accepting faith], I will give you more [of My Blessings]; but if you are thankless [i.e., ungrateful], verily My punishment is indeed severe.'" (Quran 14:7)*

Strengthening the mind-body connection

Exercise also encourages heightened awareness of the body. Islam strongly emphasises understanding the self and fostering a balanced relationship between the body and the soul.

Engaging in physical activity can help you become more aware of your body's capabilities and limitations, leading to a deeper understanding of your purpose and connection to Allah's creation.

> *The Prophet Muhammad (PBUH) said: "Your body has a right over you." (Sahih Bukhari)*

This hadith teaches that caring for your body is a religious responsibility. By exercising regularly, you honour this right and achieve greater harmony between your physical and spiritual selves.

Ritual and consistency in worship

Incorporating exercise into your daily routine can become a form of ritual that complements your spiritual practices. Just as you set aside time for prayer, fasting, and other acts of worship, dedicating time to physical exercise can provide structure and consistency in your daily life.

It serves as a reminder to prioritise both your physical and spiritual health in a balanced way.

Exercising regularly—whether it's a morning jog, a walk after prayer, or participating in a fitness routine—can serve as a spiritual ritual that keeps you grounded and connected to the purpose of your existence.

Enhancing Spiritual Fitness through Salah and Dhikr

In the hustle and bustle of daily life, it's easy to become preoccupied with the demands of work, education, social interactions, and personal responsibilities. These worldly activities can sometimes distract us from our spiritual duties and cause us to forget Allah. As our attention shifts to temporary gains, we may neglect our relationship with the Divine.

However, Allah has graciously ordained the five daily prayers (Salah) strategically placed throughout the day: in the morning, midday, late afternoon, evening, and night.

These moments of prayer serve as a powerful reminder, breaking up our routines and returning us to the core of our purpose. Praying reawakens our spiritual consciousness, redirecting our attention toward Allah and our role as His devoted servants. As stated in the Quran:

> *"And establish prayer for My remembrance." (Quran 20:14)*

Salah is not just a set of rituals; it's a continuous invitation to reconnect with Allah, reminding us of His presence and the centrality of seeking His pleasure in all aspects of our lives.

Performing Salah consistently helps nurture a deep sense of God-consciousness, known as Taqwa. With each prayer, a believer becomes more aware that Allah sees and knows everything, whether private or public. This awareness inspires a heart that is mindful of Allah's presence, fostering a delicate balance between fear of His displeasure and hope for His mercy.

Salah is a powerful motivator, encouraging Muslims to avoid sin and remain steadfast in righteousness.

> *The Quran reflects on this aspect, saying, "And be steadfast in prayer; surely, prayer restrains one from indecency and evil." (Quran 29:45)*

Through constant remembrance of Allah, a person's lifestyle becomes more aligned with divine principles. This mindfulness shapes a believer's actions, guiding them toward accountability and responsibility in Allah's sight.

It's natural for human beings to make mistakes and fall into sin. Even the most devout believers are not immune to errors, so seeking forgiveness is essential to spiritual growth. Salah provides an opportunity to turn to Allah, ask for His forgiveness, and strive for self-improvement.

Through sincere prayer, believers acknowledge their shortcomings and seek Allah's mercy. Without this regular act of repentance, a person may become desensitised to sin, gradually distancing themselves from Allah.

> *The Prophet (PBUH) beautifully explained: "What do you think if there was a river by the door of any one of you, and he bathed in it five times a day, would there be any trace of dirt left on him?" When his companions replied that no dirt would remain, the Prophet said, "That is like the five daily prayers: Allah wipes away sins through them." (Sahih Bukhari)*

Salah, therefore, not only expiates minor sins but also serves as a continual process of spiritual purification, keeping a believer constantly connected to Allah and aware of His mercy.

One of Salah's significant benefits is the discipline and self-control it fosters in believers. By praying at specific times during the day, Muslims develop a structured routine that integrates their spiritual practice with their daily activities.

Just as soldiers undergo rigorous training to develop discipline, Salah trains believers to recite specific words and perform precise physical movements while focusing their minds and hearts on Allah. Whether praying in a mosque behind an Imam or finding a quiet spot at work or school, performing Salah reinforces a sense of order and responsibility.

> *"Indeed, prayer prohibits immorality and wrongdoing..."*
> *(Quran 29:45)*

The discipline cultivated in Salah extends to other aspects of life, helping individuals avoid distractions, guard their speech, and act righteously in their interactions with others.

Another profound aspect of Salah is the peace and serenity it offers to a believer. Achieving a state of deep concentration during prayer allows the individual to experience tranquillity and humility.

> *"Successful indeed are the believers, those who humble themselves in their prayers." (Quran 23:1-2)*

Salah should not merely be a mechanical ritual but an act of devotion filled with purpose and reflection. By understanding the meanings of the Arabic words recited and contemplating the verses, believers can deepen their connection with Allah. Focusing on the words, movements, and physical postures during prayer helps establish a profound sense of closeness to the Creator.

Praying in a clean, distraction-free space, maintaining concentration, and even closing one's eyes if necessary allows the mind to focus on the worship of Allah, offering peace to the heart and mind.

The act of prostration, in particular, brings a believer closest to Allah, as the Prophet Muhammad (PBUH) said:

> *"The closest a servant comes to his Lord is when he is prostrating, so increase supplications in it." (Sahih Muslim)*

Maintaining concentration and humility during Salah requires continuous effort and practice. Spiritual highs and lows are a natural part of the believer's journey, and it's important to remain steadfast, even when prayer feels challenging. A person continuously renews their connection to Allah by persisting in Salah, allowing the prayer to transform and purify their heart and soul.

Salah is a source of inner peace, providing a spiritual retreat where the mind can reset and find solace in remembering Allah. With consistent devotion and sincerity, prayer becomes more than just a ritual; it becomes a powerful tool for spiritual growth, discipline, and serenity.

In conclusion, Salah is a key practice for enhancing spiritual fitness. It helps a believer reconnect with Allah, fosters mindfulness and discipline, promotes repentance, and provides tranquillity and serenity. Through regular prayer and sincere remembrance of Allah, a person strengthens their relationship with the Divine, aligns their actions with righteous principles, and seeks forgiveness and mercy. Salah's transformative power lies in its ability to reconnect the heart and mind to Allah, cultivating a life rooted in spiritual awareness and devotion.

The Importance of Mental Well-Being in Achieving Holistic Health

Mental well-being is a critical component of overall health and plays an essential role in the Islamic understanding of a balanced life. In Islam, health is viewed comprehensively, encompassing physical, mental, emotional, and spiritual well-being. The Quran and the teachings of the Prophet Muhammad (PBUH) guide nurturing our mental and emotional states to achieve a harmonious existence.

The Holistic View of Health in Islam

Islam emphasises a holistic approach to health and well-being, recognising that the mind, body, and soul are interconnected. A healthy mind supports a healthy body and a sound spiritual state. When mental health is neglected, it can lead to disturbances in other areas of life, ultimately affecting a person's overall well-being. The Quran encourages believers to seek balance and avoid extremes in all aspects of life:

> *"And eat and drink, but be not excessive. Indeed, He likes not those who commit excess." (Quran 7:31)*

This balance applies not only to physical health but also to maintaining emotional and psychological harmony.

Strategies for Mental Well-Being in Islam

Islam offers practical guidance for managing stress and promoting mental well-being:

Mindfulness and remembrance of Allah: Engaging in dhikr (remembrance of Allah) and mindfulness can help calm the mind and strengthen our connection with the Creator. Incorporate practices such as meditation, tasbih (repeating praises of Allah), or deep breathing exercises to manage stress.

> *"Verily, in the remembrance of Allah do hearts find rest."* (Quran 13:28)

Trust in Allah and patience (Sabr): Life comes with trials and difficulties, but placing our trust in Allah and practising patience can ease the emotional burden:

> *"And seek help through patience and prayer, and indeed, it is difficult except for the humbly submissive [to Allah]."* (Quran 2:45)

Understanding that challenges are part of life's test can help maintain emotional resilience and peace.

Maintaining hope and gratitude: The Quran encourages believers to be hopeful and grateful, focusing on the blessings in life. A grateful heart finds contentment:

> *"If you are grateful, I will surely increase you [in favour]."* (Quran 14:7)

Setting realistic goals and achieving balance: Islam advocates setting achievable goals and celebrating progress. The Prophet (PBUH) taught moderation in all matters, which helps maintain a balanced approach to personal and professional life. Believers are encouraged to set reasonable goals and make steady progress.

Mindfulness and Stress Management Techniques

In Islam, mindfulness and managing stress are deeply integrated into spiritual practices. The concept of Tafakkur (contemplation) and Muraqabah (self-vigilance) aligns with modern mindfulness, emphasising the importance of being aware of the present moment while remembering and submitting to Allah.

By practising mindfulness, Muslims can strengthen their spiritual connection and gain inner peace, helping to alleviate stress and anxiety.

What Is Mindfulness?

Mindfulness in Islam is the practice of being present, aware, and fully engaged in the current moment while remembering Allah (Dhikrullah). The Quran and the Hadiths encourage mindful awareness of one's actions, thoughts, and emotions and recognition of Allah's presence in every aspect of life.

Common Mindfulness Techniques in Islam

Several Islamic practices can help foster mindfulness and manage stress:

Mindful Breathing and Dhikr

One of the simplest mindfulness techniques involves focusing on your breath while simultaneously engaging in Dhikr, repeating praises such as "SubhanAllah" (Glory be to Allah), "Alhamdulillah" (All praise is due to Allah), and "Allahu Akbar" (Allah is the Greatest).

This exercise calms the mind, reminds us of our purpose, and strengthens our connection to Allah. Breathe deeply, letting the recitation flow with each breath, and feel the tranquillity settle in your heart.

> *"Those who have believed and whose hearts are assured by the remembrance of Allah. Unquestionably, by the remembrance of Allah hearts are assured." (Quran 13:28)*

Body Scan (Muraqabah)

While sitting or lying down, perform a body scan by focusing your attention on different parts of your body. Begin with the feet and move upwards, observing any sensations while being aware of the blessings Allah has bestowed upon your body. Avoid judgment or anxiety about discomfort; express gratitude for your physical well-being and health.

Mindful Eating with Gratitude

This practice involves eating slowly and mindfully, starting with the "Bismillah" (in the name of Allah). Pay attention to your food's colours, textures, and flavours, and be grateful for Allah's sustenance. Contemplate the source of each bite and reflect on Allah's bounty and mercy.

> *"Then eat of what Allah has provided for you [which is] lawful and good. And be grateful for the favour of Allah, if it is [indeed] Him that you worship." (Quran 16:114)*

Loving Kindness (Dua for Others)

Engage in Dua (supplication) by praying for yourself and extending prayers of peace, health, and well-being to your loved ones, acquaintances, and all of humanity. This practice fosters compassion and empathy, helping build stronger connections.

Mindful Movement and Prayer (Salah)

Perform Salah with mindfulness, being fully present in your prayer. Concentrate on each movement, the meanings of the recitations, and the act of submitting to Allah. When walking, reflect on the blessings of mobility and observe your surroundings as signs of Allah's creation.

> *"Indeed, in the creation of the heavens and the earth and the alternation of the night and the day are signs for those of understanding."(Quran 3:190)*

Stress Management Techniques in Islam

Stress and anxiety are natural parts of life, but Islam provides practical and spiritual ways to manage them:

Prayer and Sujood

One of the most effective ways to relieve stress is through Salah and placing one's head on the ground in Sujood. This act of submission to Allah brings both physical and emotional relief. The Prophet Muhammad (PBUH) said: "The closest that a servant is to his Lord is when he is in prostration."(Sahih Muslim)

Supplication and Seeking Allah's Help

Making Dua for relief from stress is a powerful tool. The Prophet (PBUH) often sought refuge from anxiety, teaching us to place our trust in Allah:

> *"O Allah, I seek refuge in You from worry and grief, helplessness and laziness, miserliness and cowardice, the burden of debts, and being overpowered by men."* (Sahih Bukhari)

Recitation of the Quran

Reading and reflecting on the Quan can bring peace and reduce stress. Verses like Ayat al-Kursi (Quran 2:255) and Surah Al-Fatihah are particularly comforting, reminding us of Allah's greatness and protection.

Trust in Allah (Tawakkul)

Placing complete trust in Allah's plan reduces anxiety about the future. Recognising that Allah is the best disposer of affairs and that He tests us only with what we can can ease the burden of stress.

> *"And whoever relies upon Allah – then He is sufficient for him." (Quran 65:3)*

Practising Gratitude

Reflecting on the blessings in your life and being grateful to Allah can uplift your spirit. Expressing gratitude helps shift your focus away from worries and onto the positives.

By adopting these Islamic mindfulness and stress management techniques, we can maintain a sense of calm, develop resilience, and achieve a harmonious balance between the mind, body, and spirit, all while deepening our connection with Allah.

Sunnah Practices for Mindfulness and Stress Relief

Islamic teachings provide various Sunnah practices that promote mindfulness and stress relief. These practices are not only spiritually uplifting but also have tangible benefits for mental well-being.

Deep Breathing and Relaxation Before Sleep

The Prophet Muhammad (PBUH) recommended specific practices to aid relaxation and prepare the mind for rest. One example is reciting

Dhikr or engaging in supplications while lying on one's right side. This practice, paired with deep breathing, calms the nervous system and reduces stress, making it easier to transition into a restful sleep.

Morning and Evening Adhkar (Remembrances)

Reciting Adhkar (plural of Dhikr) in the morning and evening is a Sunnah practice that serves as a spiritual shield against stress and anxiety. These remembrances often involve praising and thanking Allah, shifting the focus from worries to a state of gratitude and mindfulness. Repeating phrases such as "SubhanAllah" (Glory be to Allah), "Alhamdulillah" (All praise be to Allah), and "Allahu Akbar" (Allah is the Greatest) helps cultivate a sense of peace and purpose.

Seeking Solitude for Contemplation (Khalwa)

The Prophet would often seek solitude in places like the cave of Hira for reflection and meditation. This Sunnah practice emphasises taking time away from daily distractions to engage in self-reflection and spiritual connection. Engaging in quiet, contemplative moments helps believers realign their thoughts, reduce mental clutter, and find calmness amid life's stresses.

Gratitude and Positive Reframing

Expressing gratitude is a deeply embedded practice in the Sunnah. The Prophet taught the importance of focusing on blessings rather than problems. This shift in perspective can decrease stress and promote mental clarity. Gratitude exercises, like listing daily blessings or making dua (prayer) of thanks, help to foster a positive mindset and reduce the impact of negative emotions.

Structured Daily Routine with Salah (Prayer)

The five daily prayers provide structured intervals throughout the day to pause, reflect, and reset. These acts of worship involve physical postures, recitations, and moments of quiet reflection, creating natural breaks to manage stress. The routine of Salah not only enhances spiritual fitness but also fosters mindfulness, as it requires full mental presence and focus on the connection with Allah.

Techniques for Managing Stress and Promoting Mental Clarity

Mindful Breathing Techniques

Mindful breathing is one of the most effective ways to manage stress and enhance mental clarity. This technique involves taking slow, deep breaths, activating the parasympathetic nervous system and lowering stress hormones like cortisol.

Focusing on your breath also promotes present-moment awareness, which helps prevent your mind from being overwhelmed by anxious thoughts. This method can be incorporated into daily practices, especially before prayer, to prepare for a focused state of worship.

Progressive Muscle Relaxation

This technique is particularly helpful for reducing the physical tension that accompanies stress. It involves tensing and slowly relaxing different muscle groups, starting from your feet and working up to your head.

This practice not only relaxes the body but also calms the mind, fostering a sense of tranquillity. It's a valuable exercise before engaging in Salah or when feeling overwhelmed.

Visualisation and Guided Imagery

Visualisation involves mentally picturing a peaceful scene or imagining yourself successfully handling a stressful situation. This technique can redirect your focus from stressors to a place of calm, which directly reduces anxiety. Guided imagery can also be paired with Dhikr or Quranic recitation to deepen the sense of spiritual and mental calm.

Journaling for Emotional Clarity

Writing down thoughts and feelings is an effective way to declutter the mind. Journaling helps organise thoughts, identify stress triggers, and process emotions in a structured way.

The Prophet Muhammad (PBUH) emphasised self-reflection, and journaling can be seen as a modern extension of this Sunnah practice. It's a simple yet powerful tool for reducing mental stress and gaining clarity.

Mindful Engagement in Daily Activities

Mindfulness can be practised in everyday activities, such as eating, walking, or performing chores. The key is to be fully present and engaged in the moment, using all your senses to experience the task.

For example, during Wudu (ablution), you can focus on the sensation of water, the intention behind each movement, and the purification process. This mindfulness practice can transform routine activities into opportunities for mental and spiritual renewal.

Chapter Nine

Sleep Hygiene According to Sunnah

Importance of Quality Sleep in Islamic Tradition

In Islamic tradition, the importance of maintaining good physical and mental health is emphasised in many aspects of life, and quality sleep plays a vital role in this. Sleep, as a necessary component of human well-being, is not only recognised as a biological need but also as a form of worship and a means of spiritual rejuvenation.

Islam provides guidance on how to manage sleep for the benefit of both the body and the soul, encouraging balance and moderation in every aspect of life, including rest.

In Islam, sleep is viewed as a blessing from Allah (SWT). It's a natural process through which the body and mind rest, recover, and regain energy. In various verses, the Quran acknowledges sleep as a sign of Allah's creation and mercy. One such verse is:

> *"And it is He who makes [for] you the night for rest and the day for livelihood."* (Quran 25:47)

This verse highlights that the night is a time for rest and recovery, an essential part of life's cycle. Islam acknowledges that quality sleep is crucial to function effectively during the day, whether in work, worship, or family responsibilities. By recognising sleep as a divine gift, Muslims are encouraged to appreciate and manage their rest with mindfulness.

In Islam, every act, even mundane ones like eating, sleeping, or walking, can be transformed into an act of worship if done with the correct intention (niyyah). By adhering to the teachings of Islam regarding sleep, a Muslim can turn rest into an act of devotion. The Prophet Muhammad (PBUH) taught his followers that seeking rest is part of the balance that Allah has ordained for human beings. In one famous hadith, the Prophet Muhammad (PBUH) said:

> *"Your body has a right over you." (Sahih Bukhari)*

This emphasises the importance of maintaining the well-being of the body, which includes getting proper rest. The Prophet (PBUH) also recognised that excessive or insufficient sleep has negative consequences, so he encouraged moderation and balance.

The Sunnah (traditions of the Prophet) provides specific guidance on how to sleep in a way that promotes health and well-being. These practices are not merely ritualistic but founded on sound principles of maintaining a healthy lifestyle. The Prophet (PBUH) taught Muslims to sleep in specific positions, such as lying on the right side, which modern science has shown to promote better digestion and sleep quality.

> *"When you go to bed, perform ablution (wudu), then lie on your right side." (Sahih Muslim)*

This practice not only provides a physical benefit but also allows the individual to follow the Sunnah of the Prophet, turning sleep into an act of worship.

The Importance of Moderation in Sleep

Islam encourages moderation in all aspects of life, and sleep is no exception. Excess and insufficient sleep can negatively affect an individual's physical and mental health. The Prophet Muhammad (PBUH) recommended a balanced sleep schedule that included rest and waking hours, emphasising consistency. It is reported that the Prophet (PBUH) slept early, woke up early, and took a short nap (qailulah) in the afternoon.

> *"The most beloved of deeds to Allah are those which are most consistent, even if they are few." (Sahih Bukhari)*

This hadith emphasises the importance of consistency, even in sleep. A regular, balanced sleep schedule allows the body to function optimally. A good night's sleep, in alignment with the Sunnah, ensures that an individual wakes up refreshed and able to engage in daily activities with full energy. This, in turn, increases one's ability to worship and serve others.

The benefits of sleep in Islam are not only physical but also spiritual. Restful sleep allows a person to be more productive in their daily tasks, more present in their prayers, and better able to fulfil their religious obligations. Muslims who get adequate rest are also better equipped to practice self-control, avoid excessive anger, and manage stress. In fact, quality sleep can improve an individual's overall mental health, which is vital for personal development and well-being.

Sleep is essential for mental clarity, which allows a person to think critically, make sound decisions, and manage life's challenges. The

Quran underscores the importance of maintaining a healthy mind and body, as both are vital for fulfilling the role of a servant of Allah.

> *"And We have certainly created man, and We know what his soul whispers to him, and We are closer to him than [his] jugular vein." (Quran 50:16)*

This verse demonstrates that Allah is deeply concerned with human well-being, both physically and spiritually. Rest and sleep are part of this divine care, ensuring that individuals are physically rested and mentally sharp to fulfil their purpose.

In addition to its health benefits, sleep has spiritual dimensions in Islam. For example, Muslims are encouraged to recite specific prayers (duas) before sleeping, such as the Ayat-ul-Kursi (Quran, 2:255), to seek protection from harm during the night. By invoking the name of Allah before sleep, the believer is assured of divine protection and peace of mind during rest.

The Prophet Muhammad (PBUH) also taught that sleep is a way for the soul to refresh and rejuvenate itself. A well-rested person is more likely to pray with focus and devotion, leading to a stronger connection with Allah.

In conclusion, sleep in Islam is not merely a biological necessity but a means of maintaining overall physical and spiritual well-being. Quality sleep is acknowledged as a blessing from Allah, and following the practices outlined in the Quran and Sunnah can turn sleep into an act of worship. Balancing rest with productivity and following the guidance of the Prophet Muhammad (PBUH) on sleep ensures Muslims a healthy, fulfilling life according to their faith. As with all aspects of life, Islam teaches moderation, mindfulness, and the importance of self-care, which is essential for maintaining the body's vitality and the soul's tranquillity.

Prophetic Guidance on Sleep Hygiene and its Benefits

The Prophet Muhammad (PBUH) imparted clear and practical wisdom on achieving restful and rejuvenating sleep. His teachings on sleep hygiene focused on the physical aspects of sleep and addressed spiritual and mental well-being, recognising that proper rest is crucial for the body and the soul. This prophetic guidance is timeless, offering practical advice that remains relevant today.

1. Sleeping early and waking early

One of the most notable aspects of the Prophet's (PBUH) sleep habits was his routine of sleeping early and waking early. Islam encourages Muslims to adopt a productive lifestyle, reflected in the Prophet's schedule. He would sleep soon after the Isha (night) prayer and wake up early before Fajr (dawn) to perform the Tahajjud (night prayer). This practice ensures a person gets enough rest and ample time for worship and productive activities during the day.

> *The Prophet (PBUH) said: "O 'Abd al-Rahman ibn Qudama! If you can, do not sleep except at night, and do not stay up except at night." (Sunan Tirmidhi)*

This guidance emphasises the importance of a clear division between sleep and wakefulness, ensuring that sleep happens in harmony with the natural rhythms of the day.

2. The Sunnah of sleeping on the right side

The Prophet (PBUH) instructed Muslims to sleep on their right side, as the most beneficial for the body and the soul. In addition to being the Sunnah of the Prophet, this position has also been scientifically linked to better digestion and circulation. The Prophet (PBUH) said: "When you go to bed, perform ablution (wudu), then lie on your right side."(Sahih Muslim) This recommendation is significant for physical comfort and spiritual alignment, as sleeping in this way helps prepare an individual for a peaceful and blessed night.

3. Performing Wudu (Ablution) before sleeping

Another important aspect of sleep hygiene in Islam is performing wudu (ablution) before sleeping. Wudu is a form of purification that prepares the individual for rest and spiritual peace. It is narrated that the Prophet (PBUH) would perform wudu before sleeping, stating:

> *"Purify yourself, for it is a means of protection for you."*
> *(Sahih Bukhari)*

This practice not only enhances cleanliness but also helps the person feel spiritually refreshed and ready for sleep, with the added benefit of invoking the protection of Allah during the night.

4. Reciting specific Duas and verses before sleep

The Prophet Muhammad (PBUH) taught specific prayers and Quranic verses to recite before bed to ensure peace, protection, and blessings during sleep.

One of the most well-known supplications is the recitation of Ayat-ul-Kursi, which is said to offer protection from harm:

> *"Allah! There is no deity except Him, the Ever-Living, the Sustainer of existence..." (Quran 2:255)*

Reciting this verse before sleep helps ensure that the individual is spiritually protected and able to sleep peacefully. The Prophet (PBUH) also recommended reciting the last two verses of Surah Al-Baqarah before bed, which provide a sense of comfort and security:

> *"Allah does not burden a soul beyond that it can bear"*
> *(Quran 2:286)*

These verses remind believers of Allah's mercy and care, contributing to a calm and restful sleep.

Islam strongly emphasises cleanliness, which extends to the area where a person sleeps. The Prophet (PBUH) instructed that the sleeping area should be kept clean and impurities-free. It is reported that the Prophet (PBUH) said:

> *"When one of you goes to sleep, let him tidy his bed and shake it out, for he does not know what might have entered it."* (Sahih Bukhari)

This practice ensures cleanliness and promotes mental clarity, as a clean and organised environment is conducive to peaceful sleep.

While Islam encourages rest, the Prophet (PBUH) also cautioned against excessive sleep, as it can lead to laziness and neglect of important duties. The Prophet (PBUH) said:

> *"Do not make your sleep too long, for it will make you lazy and neglectful of worship."* (Sunan Ibn Majah)

Excessive sleep leads to a lack of productivity and can interfere with one's ability to engage in acts of worship, family responsibilities, and personal growth. Thus, the Prophet (PBUH) recommended a balanced approach, ensuring sleep does not hinder one's daily obligations.

The Prophet (PBUH) also advocated for a short nap in the afternoon, known as qailulah. This practice is recommended to restore energy and improve alertness for the rest of the day. It is narrated that the Prophet (PBUH) would take a short nap after the Dhuhr prayer, which allowed him to remain active and energised for the evening:

> *"Take a nap, for indeed the devils do not take a nap."*
> *(Sahih Bukhari)*

Taking a brief nap, especially in the early afternoon, has both physical and spiritual benefits. Scientific studies have shown that it improves cognitive function, enhances memory, and boosts overall productivity.

Finally, the Prophet (PBUH) encouraged gratitude for the gift of sleep. In a beautiful supplication, the Prophet (PBUH) would thank Allah for providing him with rest each night:

> *"O Allah, I have submitted myself to You, and I have turned my face to You, and I have entrusted my affairs to You." (Sahih Muslim)*

This prayer expresses gratitude for the rest that Allah (SWT) provides and reminds us that sleep is a gift not to be taken for granted. By recognising the blessing of sleep, we can elevate resting to an act of worship.

The Prophet Muhammad's (PBUH) guidance on sleep hygiene offers a holistic approach that includes physical, mental, and spiritual aspects. By following these practices, Muslims can maintain a balanced and healthy sleep routine that promotes physical well-being and strengthens their relationship with Allah.

Quality sleep is essential for a productive, fulfilling life, and the prophetic teachings serve as a timeless guide for achieving rest that benefits both body and soul.

Tips for Improving Sleep Quality: A Guide to Better Rest through Islamic Principles

Sleep is vital to our lives, affecting our physical health, mental well-being, and overall productivity. In Islam, the significance of sleep is acknowledged and emphasised as an essential part of a balanced life.

The Quran and Hadith provide valuable insights into the importance of sleep and how we can improve its quality. The following section will cover tips for improving sleep quality grounded in Islamic teachings, including creating a conducive sleep environment, adhering to Sunnah bedtime practices, and using relaxation techniques.

Creating a conducive sleep environment (Nuzul al-Mu'min)

The environment in which we sleep plays a critical role in the quality of our rest. In Islam, there is guidance on creating a peaceful and comfortable space for sleep. The term Nuzul al-Mu'min can be understood as preparing a restful space for believers to rejuvenate their bodies and souls.

A good sleep environment is one that is quiet, clean, and comfortable. As mentioned, Islam encourages cleanliness and orderliness in all aspects of life, including the sleeping area. The Prophet Muhammad (PBUH) emphasised the importance of cleanliness, and this advice stands even in the context of sleep.

> *"Cleanliness is half of faith." (Sahih Muslim)*

To create an optimal sleep environment, consider the following elements:

Clean and tidy space: The bed and sleeping area should be clean, as cleanliness fosters a peaceful state of mind. In the Quran, Allah (SWT) commands believers to maintain cleanliness:

"Indeed, Allah loves those who are constantly repentant and loves those who purify themselves." (Quran 2:222)

A clean and well-kept space contributes to relaxation and promotes better sleep.

Temperature control: In Islam, avoiding sleeping in extremes of heat or cold is recommended. The Prophet Muhammad (PBUH) advised moderation in all aspects of life, including temperature. Sleeping at a comfortable and balanced temperature can prevent discomfort during the night and aid in restful sleep.

Minimise distractions: To create a conducive environment for sleep, limit distractions such as noise and light. The Prophet (PBUH) recommended minimising distractions before sleep by making dua (supplication) and engaging in dhikr (remembrance of Allah) to calm the mind.

Chapter Ten

Hydration and Sunnah Drinking Habits

Hydration is essential for maintaining good health, and the significance of drinking water is emphasised in many religious and cultural traditions, including Islam.

The teachings of the Prophet Muhammad (PBUH) provide valuable insights into the importance of staying hydrated and specific guidelines on how to drink water in a way that benefits both the body and the soul.

In this section, we'll explore the importance of staying hydrated according to Islamic teachings and the prophetic traditions related to drinking water and its health benefits.

Importance of Staying Hydrated According to Islamic Teachings

Water is considered one of the greatest blessings from Allah (SWT) in Islam. The Quran repeatedly mentions water as a sign of Allah's mercy and sustenance.

In several verses, Allah emphasises the role of water in sustaining life and nourishing the earth:

> *"And We made from water every living thing. Then will they not believe?" (Quran 21:30)*

This verse highlights that water is essential not only for the physical survival of living beings but also as a reminder of Allah's infinite power and provision. Hydration is, therefore, not just a physical need but also a spiritual reminder to be grateful for Allah's blessings.

Water as a Source of Health and Life

The Quran also emphasises that water is a source of life, vital for the growth of plants and the prosperity of civilisation. It is a fundamental resource that enables crops, animals, and humans to thrive:

> *"And We sent down from the sky blessed water, that We may bring forth thereby fruits and vegetables, and grain and the crops." (Quran 50:9)*

The significance of water in Islam is not limited to survival but extends to the well-being of the individual. Staying hydrated is, therefore, a means of taking care of one's body, which is considered a trust (Amanah) from Allah. As the Prophet Muhammad (PBUH) said:

> *"Your body has a right over you." (Sahih Bukhari)*

This Hadith underscores the profound responsibility of caring for the body, a trust bestowed by Allah. It highlights that maintaining health and well-being – including something as fundamental as staying hydrated – is not just a personal duty but a spiritual act of stewardship.

Prophetic Traditions Related to Drinking Water and Its Health Benefits

The Prophet Muhammad (PBUH) provided clear and detailed guidance on drinking water, promoting habits that benefit both the body and the soul. His instructions go beyond simple hydration, emphasising moderation, gratitude, and mindfulness in the act of drinking.

One of the most important guidelines provided by the Prophet (PBUH) is to drink water in small sips rather than gulping large quantities at once. This is not only beneficial for digestion but also encourages mindfulness while drinking. The Prophet (PBUH) said:

> *"Do not drink water in one gulp like a camel, but drink in two or three sips."(Sunan Tirmidhi)*

Drinking in sips gives the body time to absorb the water gradually, aiding in better hydration and reducing the risk of indigestion. This practice also promotes a more peaceful and meditative approach to daily actions. Another key guideline from the Sunnah is to drink water while sitting rather than standing. The Prophet (PBUH) instructed:

> *"Do not drink while standing." (Sahih Muslim)*

Drinking while seated is not only a recommendation for proper etiquette but also promotes better digestion and water absorption. Modern medical science supports this, suggesting that sitting while drinking helps relax the body and ensures water flows properly through the digestive system.

Islam teaches gratitude in every action, and drinking water is no exception. The Prophet Muhammad (PBUH) recommended saying a short supplication before and after drinking water to acknowledge the blessing of hydration. He said:

> *"When you drink, say Bismillah (In the name of Allah), and when you finish, say Alhamdulillah (All praise is due to Allah)." (Sunan Tirmidhi)*

This simple act of gratitude helps remind the believer of Allah's (SWT) mercy in providing sustenance. It also elevates the mundane act of drinking water into an act of worship and mindfulness. The Prophet (PBUH) recommended drinking water after waking up, emphasising the importance of starting the day with hydration.

> *"The two rak'ahs before dawn, and the two sips of water after waking up in the morning are a remedy for every ailment." (Sunan al-Kubra)*

Drinking water after waking up helps to replenish fluids lost during the night and jump-starts the body's metabolism. It also helps clear toxins from the body, providing a natural form of detoxification and boosting energy levels.

While staying hydrated is essential, Islam also teaches moderation in all aspects of life, including water consumption. The Prophet Muhammad (PBUH) encouraged balance in all habits, including drinking:

> *"The son of Adam does not fill any vessel worse than his stomach. It is sufficient for the son of Adam to eat a few mouthfuls to keep his back straight. If he must eat more, then let him fill one-third with food, one-third with drink, and one-third with air." (Sunan Ibn Majah)*

This Hadith emphasises that overconsumption, even of something as vital as water, can harm the body. Drinking in moderation ensures the body remains balanced and healthy rather than overwhelmed or sluggish from excess.

In Islamic tradition, drinking water is not only a physical necessity but also linked to numerous health benefits. The Prophet Muhammad (PBUH) was aware of water's healing properties and used it for various health-related purposes, including hydration and therapy.

"Water is the best drink." (Sahih Bukhari)

This highlights the universal and timeless recognition of water's healing properties. In modern times, water is recognised for its role in maintaining body temperature, supporting digestion, and promoting overall health. Islam's emphasis on water aligns with contemporary understandings of its essential role in bodily functions.

Hydration is a fundamental aspect of health, and Islam provides a comprehensive framework for ensuring that we drink water in a way that benefits both our physical bodies and spiritual well-being.

The prophetic guidelines on hydration—such as drinking in small sips, sitting while drinking, showing gratitude, and maintaining moderation—are not just health recommendations but are an integral part of the Islamic way of life.

Following these Sunnah practices, we can cultivate a holistic approach to hydration grounded in mindfulness, gratitude, and balance. These practices enhance our health, deepen our spiritual connection with Allah (SWT), and promote well-being for both body and soul.

Drinking water in the prescribed manner is not just a physical necessity; it is an act of worship that nourishes our bodies and souls alike.

Health Benefits of Sunnah Beverages

Certain beverages hold unique significance in Islamic tradition due to their spiritual and health benefits. These beverages, such as Zamzam water, are not only seen as a means of hydration but also as gifts from Allah (SWT) with profound blessings and healing properties.

Incorporating Sunnah beverages into our daily hydration routines is a way to align our health practices with the teachings of the Prophet Muhammad (PBUH) while also gaining spiritual rewards.

This section will explore the health benefits of Sunnah beverages, specifically Zamzam water, and provide tips for maintaining optimal hydration throughout the day, drawing from Islamic traditions.

Incorporating Sunnah Beverages into Daily Hydration Routines

Zamzam water holds a unique and revered status in Islam. It's drawn from the sacred Zamzam Well, located in the Masjid al-Haram in Mecca and is believed to have been miraculously provided by Allah for Hajar (the wife of Prophet Ibrahim) and their son Ismail (PBUH) centuries ago.

The significance of Zamzam water is not only spiritual but also believed to have remarkable health benefits.

> *The Prophet Muhammad (PBUH) said: "Zamzam water is for whatever it is drunk for." (Sahih Muslim)*

This Hadith highlights the profound nature of Zamzam water. It's not merely water but a source of blessings, healing, and fulfilment of specific needs. Whether consumed for physical health, seeking blessings, or spiritual intentions, Zamzam water has a unique place in Islamic tradition. Many Muslims drink Zamzam water during pilgrimage, and it is often believed to bring about positive changes in one's health, spiritual state, and even the fulfilment of one's wishes.

From a health perspective, Zamzam water has been studied for its mineral content. The water contains a high concentration of essential minerals, such as calcium, magnesium, and sodium, which help in rehydration, boosting energy, and maintaining body functions.

Studies have shown that Zamzam water is pure, free from contaminants, and has a balanced mineral composition, making it beneficial for the body to maintain hydration and support overall health.

Another important beverage the Prophet Muhammad (PBUH) recommended for health benefits is honey mixed with water. Honey, as described in the Quran, is a source of healing:

> *"And your Lord inspired the bee, saying, 'Take for yourself among the mountains, houses, and among the trees and in which they plant. Then eat from all the fruits and follow the ways of your Lord laid down for you.' There emerges from their bellies a drink of varying colours, in which there is healing for people." (Quran 16:68-69)*

The Prophet (PBUH) also recommended honey for its health benefits, saying:

> *"Make use of medical treatment, for Allah has not made a disease without appointing a remedy for it, with the exception of old age." (Sahih al-Bukhari)*

Honey mixed with warm water can provide numerous health benefits, including aiding digestion, strengthening the immune system, and offering natural antimicrobial properties. Drinking this Sunnah beverage in the morning or before meals can enhance digestion and help detoxify the body.

Milk is another beverage praised in Islam for its health benefits. The Prophet Muhammad (PBUH) enjoyed drinking milk and recommended it for its nourishing qualities. He said:

> *"There is no drink more beneficial than milk." (Sahih Muslim)*

Milk is rich in essential nutrients, such as calcium, vitamin D, and protein, making it a wholesome beverage for maintaining strong bones, teeth, and muscles. Consuming milk in moderation can also help improve digestion and overall vitality.

Incorporating Sunnah Beverages into Daily Hydration Routines

To integrate Sunnah beverages into your daily hydration routine, it is important to maintain consistency and balance. Here are some practical tips for including these beverages in your diet:

Start your day with Zamzam water: If you have access to Zamzam water, make it a habit to start your day by drinking a small glass of it. According to the Sunnah, water, in general, should be drunk in sips, so begin your morning with a few small sips of Zamzam water. The Prophet Muhammad (PBUH) said:

> *"The best of the drink is that which is drunk in sips." (Sahih Muslim)*

Starting the day with Zamzam water, especially with the intention of seeking blessings and good health, is a spiritually uplifting way to begin your day.

Honey and water for digestive health: Incorporate honey mixed with warm water into your morning routine. A teaspoon of pure honey in warm water is a great way to boost your energy, aid digestion, and enjoy honey's healing properties. This practice aligns with the Sunnah and provides health benefits that support your digestive system, help detoxify your body, and offer a natural energy boost.

Drink milk for nourishment and strength: Consider drinking milk as part of your daily hydration routine, especially as a source of nourishment. You can drink it in the morning, as part of breakfast, or in the evening before bedtime for better sleep. Milk's nourishing properties, particularly its calcium and vitamin D content, make it a great addition to your hydration routine, supporting bone health and overall vitality.

Tips for Maintaining Optimal Hydration Throughout the Day

While incorporating Sunnah beverages into your routine is beneficial, it is also important to maintain hydration throughout the day. Here are some tips to ensure you're consistently hydrated:

Drink water in moderation: Islam encourages moderation in all things, including water consumption. The Prophet Muhammad (PBUH) advised drinking water in moderation, stating that the stomach should not be overly filled with food or drink. This practice helps the body maintain balance and prevents overhydration.

Drink water throughout the day in small sips rather than large gulps. Keep a water bottle nearby, and aim to drink water regularly to stay hydrated. If fasting during Ramadan, drink plenty of water during suhoor (pre-dawn meal) and iftar (meal to break the fast).

Avoid sugary or caffeinated drinks: While it is important to stay hydrated, it is best to avoid sugary or highly caffeinated beverages that can lead to dehydration. Stick to water, milk, and Sunnah beverages like honey water, as they are more beneficial for hydration and overall health.

Increase hydration with fruits and vegetables: Another natural way to stay hydrated is by incorporating fruits and vegetables with high water content into your diet. Cucumbers, watermelons, oranges, and strawberries are perfect examples of hydrating foods that provide essential nutrients and contribute to overall hydration.

Incorporating Sunnah beverages into your daily hydration routine offers numerous physical, spiritual, and health benefits. Drinking Zamzam water, honey mixed with water, and milk will align you with the practices of the Prophet Muhammad (PBUH) and benefit from the blessings and nourishment they provide.

Staying hydrated is not only a matter of physical health but also a means of seeking Allah's (SWT) blessings and following the Sunnah in our everyday lives. Through mindful consumption of these Sunnah beverages and maintaining a balanced hydration routine, we can support our health, enhance our well-being, and foster a deeper connection with the teachings of Islam.

Chapter Eleven

Implementing Sunnah Nutrition and Fitness Principles

Islam is not merely focused on worship and preparing for the Hereafter; it also encourages its followers to live a happy life – mentally, physically and spiritually – in this world. The Quran and the hadith highlight the importance of looking after oneself.

"Your body has a right over you" (Sahih Bukhari)

This succinct yet deeply meaningful narration sums up the need to keep ourselves in good health. Our bodies are an Amanah (trust) from Allah (SWT), and health is a blessing, making it imperative for us to look after ourselves but in a manner that is within the bounds of Islam.

As spoken about in-depth in an earlier section of the book, the consumption of food and drink in Islamic legal terms can be divided into what is allowed (halal) and what is forbidden (haram).

Halal is an Arabic word meaning 'lawful' or 'permissible'. The opposite of halal is haram, which means 'unlawful' or 'forbidden.' According to Islamic law, *"all foods are considered halal, or lawful, except for pork* and its by-products, animals improperly slaughtered or dead before slaughtering, animals slaughtered in the name of anyone but Allah (God), carnivorous animals, birds of prey, animals without external ears (some birds and reptiles), blood, alcohol, and foods contaminated with any of these."

Halal food is a command from Allah (SWT), and those items that are halal are permitted for consumption.

> "Eat of what is lawful and wholesome on the earth." (Quran 2:168)

In general terms, halal food items include:

- All fruits, vegetables and grains, except those that cause intoxication.
- All beef, poultry, and lamb products slaughtered according to Islamic dietary laws.
- All vegetable ingredients, except those that cause intoxication.

Haram (forbidden) foods involve pork, crustaceans, blood, and non-halal animal additives, including gelatin or suet, alcohol, and any food containing alcohol.

> "So eat of that (meat) upon which Allah's name has been mentioned if you are believers in His verses" (Quran 6:118)

> "And do not eat that upon which the name of Allah has not been mentioned, for indeed it is a grave disobedience" (Quran 6:121)

For the animals allowed for consumption, the Islamic Shariah prescribes a specific method for animal slaughter (Zabihah), which includes reciting Bismillah and Takbir and slaughtering the animal painlessly.

Herbivores and cud-chewing animals like cattle, deer, sheep, goats, and antelope are some examples of halal animals. Milk and dairy products are also considered halal.

Food items that are haram include alcohol, pork, carrion, the meat of carnivores, and animals that died due to illness, injury, stunning, poisoning, or slaughtering not in the name of Allah (SWT).

Apart from laying down rules for the lawfulness of food and drink, Islam has also highlighted certain etiquettes for dining, eating and drinking. The Prophet (PBUH) has strongly advised that one should wash his hands before and after a meal.

> *"Whoever would like to increase the goodness of his house, should perform ablution (wash hands) when his breakfast is brought to him and when it is taken away." (Sunan Ibn Majah)*

Muslims are also advised to recite specific duas before and after a meal to ensure Barakah. Another important guideline for dining and food is to cover food containers before sleeping at night.

> *"Extinguish the lamps when you go to bed; close your doors; tie the mouths of your water skins, and cover the food and drinks." I think he added, "... even with a stick you place across the container." (Sahih Bukhari)*

Practical Steps for Living a Sunnah-Based Lifestyle

Creating a personalised nutrition and fitness plan based on Sunnah principles

Living a Sunnah-based lifestyle involves adopting the teachings and practices of Prophet Muhammad (PBUH) in all aspects of life, including health, nutrition, and fitness. The Sunnah offers timeless wisdom that balances spiritual, mental, and physical well-being. In today's world, this can be a meaningful guide to creating a personalised nutrition and fitness plan that aligns with Islamic principles.

By incorporating the Sunnah's emphasis on moderation, balance, and mindfulness, you can cultivate a lifestyle that promotes not only physical health but also spiritual growth.

One of the core principles of Sunnah nutrition is eating in moderation. The Prophet (PBUH) often emphasised the importance of not overeating, saying,

> *"The son of Adam does not fill any vessel worse than his stomach. It is sufficient for the son of Adam to eat a few mouthfuls to keep him going." (Tirmidhi)*

This highlights the importance of portion control, which can be particularly helpful in the modern world, where overeating has become common. To create a personalised nutrition plan based on this principle, start by practising mindful eating.

Focus on eating slowly and stopping when you feel satisfied, not full. This approach encourages self-control, prevents excessive consumption, and allows the body time to signal when it has had enough.

In addition to moderation, the Sunnah emphasises balance in nutrition. The Prophet (PBUH) encouraged eating a variety of foods, including grains, fruits, vegetables, and lean meats, ensuring a well-rounded and nutritious diet. For instance, the Prophet (PBUH) commonly consumed dates and honey for their natural energy-boosting properties. Olive oil, also favoured by the Prophet (PBUH), is rich in healthy fats and antioxidants. Including these in your diet can not only enhance your health but also follow the Sunnah's approach to food.

A balanced diet is not just about variety but also about the proportions of each food group. Aim for meals that include complex carbohydrates like whole grains, lean proteins such as chicken or fish, healthy fats from sources like olive oil or nuts, and a variety of vegetables for vitamins and minerals. Ensuring that each meal is balanced will nourish your body in a way that supports both physical and mental energy.

Another important aspect of nutrition in the Sunnah is hydration. The Prophet (PBUH) recommended drinking water in moderation, taking three sips rather than gulping large amounts all at once. He also advised drinking with the right hand, a practice that promotes mindfulness. To integrate this into your routine, make it a habit to drink water slowly and consciously, remembering to say "Bismillah" before drinking and "Alhamdulillah" afterwards.

By following these practices, not only are you staying hydrated, but you're also cultivating gratitude and mindfulness with every sip. You may also incorporate drinks such as Zamzam water or natural herbal teas, frequently consumed by the Prophet (PBUH), further enriching your nutrition plan.

Fasting is another vital element of the Sunnah that has numerous health benefits. The Prophet (PBUH) regularly fasted on Mondays and Thursdays, a practice that has spiritual significance as well as health benefits. Fasting allows the digestive system to rest, promotes detoxification, and can contribute to mental clarity. For a personalised approach, consider fasting on the days recommended in the Sunnah, or if that isn't feasible, try intermittent fasting. Start with smaller fasting periods, gradually building your tolerance while ensuring that your meals are balanced and nutritious when you do eat. This could include a nutritious pre-dawn meal (suhoor) and a wholesome iftar (meal to break the fast), incorporating a variety of fruits, vegetables, proteins, and healthy fats, as recommended in the Sunnah.

Fitness in the Sunnah is equally important, as physical health was a priority for the Prophet (PBUH). The Prophet (PBUH) was known for his active lifestyle, regularly engaging in physical activities like walking, horseback riding, archery, and swimming. These activities not only promote strength and endurance but also help maintain mental clarity and emotional balance. To create a personalised fitness plan, consider incorporating a variety of these exercises into your routine. If horseback riding or archery isn't practical for you, try cycling or joining a sports team, both of which are excellent for building coordination and cardiovascular health.

Walking is one of the most straightforward and beneficial forms of exercise mentioned in the Sunnah. The Prophet (PBUH) often walked to different places, including the mosque, which shows the importance of incorporating walking into your daily routine. Walking can help reduce stress, improve circulation, and enhance mental clarity. Aim to walk for at least 30 minutes a day. Over time, you can increase the duration and intensity.

Strength training is another important aspect of fitness in the Sunnah, even though the Prophet (PBUH) didn't specifically mention modern weightlifting techniques. However, he practised activities that built strength, such as carrying heavy loads and helping with household tasks. Consider bodyweight exercises like push-ups, squats, and planks. These exercises don't require equipment and can be done at home. You can also incorporate weight training or resistance bands into your workout routine if you prefer a more structured approach. The key is to focus on building functional strength, just as the Prophet (PBUH) did in his daily activities.

The practice of Salah, the five daily prayers, is also an integral form of physical exercise. The movements in prayer—standing, bowing, and prostrating—help improve flexibility, balance, and circulation. Performing Salah with full attention and proper posture maximises the physical benefits of these movements. Focusing on these movements during prayer enhances both spiritual and physical well-being.

Integrating these Sunnah-based nutrition and fitness principles into your daily life can significantly improve your health and well-being. Start by incorporating small changes into your routine, such as practising mindful eating, walking daily, drinking water slowly, and gradually building up to fasting and exercising regularly.

By making these practices a part of your lifestyle, you'll not only follow the example set by the Prophet (PBUH) but also experience the numerous benefits to your physical, mental, and spiritual health. With consistency, patience, and mindfulness, you can live a fulfilling life aligned with the Sunnah's teachings.

Overcoming Challenges and Integrating Sunnah Practices into Daily Life

Integrating Sunnah practices into daily life can bring numerous benefits to our physical, mental, and spiritual well-being, but it often comes with challenges, especially in the context of modern, fast-paced living. The teachings and practices of Prophet Muhammad (PBUH) offer timeless wisdom that, when properly incorporated, can enhance our daily routines.

However, obstacles such as time constraints, social pressures, and lifestyle habits can make it difficult to consistently adopt these practices. Below are some common challenges and practical strategies for overcoming them to integrate Sunnah practices into your daily life effectively.

One of the most common challenges is time management. In today's world, people often feel overwhelmed with work, family commitments, and social obligations, leaving little time for religious or health practices. This can make it difficult to regularly perform acts like prayer, fasting, or eating in moderation as prescribed in the Sunnah.

A practical solution to this challenge is planning and scheduling. The key to overcoming time constraints is prioritising and setting aside specific times for Sunnah practices. For example, set a routine for Salah (prayers) by creating reminders or alarms. The five daily prayers are opportunities to reconnect with Allah (SWT) and can serve as natural breaks in your day, offering a chance to pause, reflect, and rejuvenate. Ensuring that these prayers are a priority creates space for them, even within a busy schedule.

Similarly, incorporating Sunnah-based nutrition and fitness helps to set a realistic, flexible schedule. Instead of overloading yourself with the expectation of making drastic changes, start with small, manageable steps. Begin by dedicating time for a 10-minute walk after each prayer or integrating moderate portion control into your meals. Gradually, these actions will become habits, and you'll find they fit naturally into your daily life.

Another challenge many face is maintaining consistency. Adopting new habits requires dedication, and people often struggle to stay consistent, especially when they don't see immediate results. This challenge can be particularly evident when trying to maintain Sunnah fasting (e.g., fasting on Mondays and Thursdays) or sticking to a balanced diet. The initial enthusiasm may fade, and a lack of motivation can set in.

To overcome this, set achievable goals and track progress. Breaking down larger goals into smaller, more attainable milestones can make the journey feel less overwhelming. For instance, instead of committing to fasting every week right away, begin by fasting once a month, then gradually increase the frequency. Tracking your progress and acknowledging small successes will boost your morale and keep you on track. Surrounding yourself with a supportive community or family members who practice Sunnah can also provide motivation. This social reinforcement helps keep you consistent, as accountability to others can be a powerful motivator.

Social pressures and modern lifestyle influences present another significant obstacle. In contemporary society, unhealthy eating habits, sedentary lifestyles, and negative social influences often work against the Sunnah practices. Whether it's the temptation to eat unhealthy foods or the societal emphasis on convenience over health, these external pressures can lead to challenges in adhering to Sunnah principles.

One way to overcome this is by creating a supportive environment. Try to surround yourself with people who share similar goals or support your efforts to live a Sunnah-based lifestyle. If you're working towards a Sunnah diet, seek out local communities or online groups where you can share experiences, recipes, and tips. When eating out, consider choosing healthier, Sunnah-compliant options such as meals with lean meats, vegetables, and dates. If you face temptations, remember the teachings of the Prophet (PBUH), who advocated for self-restraint and discipline, and use those moments as opportunities to practice patience.

Additionally, to counter sedentary behaviour, consider incorporating physical activity into your daily routine in a natural and manageable way. For example, walking to the mosque for prayer, taking the stairs instead of the elevator, or participating in family activities like sports or outdoor walks can provide simple yet effective ways to stay active while following the Sunnah.

Another challenge is adjusting to new practices in a modern setting, especially with aspects of the Sunnah that may not be as easily incorporated into a busy lifestyle. For example, engaging in physical activities like horseback riding, swimming, or archery, which the Prophet (PBUH) recommended, may not be practical for everyone today due to lack of facilities or time.

In this case, it's important to remember the essence behind these practices. The Prophet emphasised staying active and engaging in exercises that build strength, coordination, and mental clarity. While you may not have access to horseback riding or archery, you can replace them with other activities that offer similar benefits. Cycling, running, swimming, or practising yoga can provide cardiovascular benefits and help build strength, just as the physical activities of the Prophet (PBUH) did. The key is finding activities you enjoy that align with the Sunnah's emphasis on maintaining a healthy body.

Lastly, maintaining mindfulness and gratitude can sometimes be overlooked when integrating Sunnah practices into daily life. It's easy to become so focused on tasks and routines that we forget the deeper spiritual aspect of these practices. For instance, eating with your right hand, drinking in moderation, or saying "Bismillah" before meals should not be seen as just tasks to check off but as moments to cultivate gratitude and mindfulness.

To address this challenge, it's important to slow down and be present in each moment. When you drink water or eat, take a moment to reflect on the blessings of food, water, and health and make a conscious effort to incorporate the Sunnah's mindfulness into your actions. Similarly, during your daily prayers, focus on the connection you're building with Allah (SWT) and the peace it brings rather than simply completing a ritual.

Incorporating Sunnah practices into daily life is a gradual process, and it requires patience, intention, and persistence. The key to overcoming challenges is not perfection but continuous effort and striving to align your life with the teachings of the Prophet (PBUH). By setting realistic goals, finding support, and being consistent, you can create a balanced and fulfilling lifestyle that honours the Sunnah and enhances your overall well-being. Through these efforts, you not only improve your physical health but also draw closer to Allah (SWT) and lead a life full of purpose and meaning.

Embracing Health and Well-being through Sunnah Practices

In a world where fast-paced lifestyles and modern conveniences often lead to unhealthy habits, it's essential to pause and reflect on timeless wisdom. One such source of wisdom is the Sunnah, the way of life taught by the Prophet (PBUH), which encourages a holistic approach to health, encompassing not just the physical but also the mental, emotional, and spiritual dimensions of well-being. By integrating the teachings of the Sunnah into our daily routines, we can nurture a balanced and mindful approach to nutrition, fitness, and overall health.

Inspiring a Balanced and Mindful Approach to Nutrition, Fitness, and Overall Well-being

The Sunnah emphasises moderation in all aspects of life, including nutrition and physical activity. Prophet Muhammad (PBUH) taught us to consume food in a balanced manner, focusing on nourishment rather than indulgence. In the famous Hadith, he encouraged eating in moderation, saying:

> *"The son of Adam does not fill any vessel worse than his stomach; it is enough for him to eat a few mouthfuls that will keep his back straight." (Sunan Ibn Majah)*

This teaches us the importance of mindful eating – being conscious of portion sizes, enjoying meals in gratitude, and avoiding excess. Islamic dietary guidelines also emphasise the consumption of wholesome foods that promote health, such as fruits, vegetables, whole grains, and lean proteins, while advising against harmful substances like alcohol and excessive consumption of processed foods.

Physical fitness is equally valued in the Sunnah. The Prophet (PBUH) encouraged physical activity, from walking to practising archery, swimming, and horseback riding. He even referred to archery as a form of "training" for both body and mind. Regular physical activity, in line with the Sunnah, enhances physical strength, mental clarity, and emotional resilience, which are key components of overall well-being.

Committing to Lifelong Health Habits Rooted in Islamic Teachings and Prophetic Traditions

Health, according to the teachings of Islam, is a trust from Allah (SWT), and we're encouraged to maintain it as a lifelong commitment.

> *"There are two blessings which many people lose: health and free time." (Sahih Bukhari)*

This reminder prompts us to not only appreciate the health we have but also take proactive steps to maintain it.

A commitment to lifelong health is not a one-time decision but a continuous process. The Sunnah encourages consistent habits, such as regular prayer, which includes physical movements that promote flexibility, balance, and circulation. Fasting during Ramadan also provides physical and spiritual benefits, offering a time to detoxify, reflect, and develop self-discipline.

Islam encourages holistic self-care, ensuring we prioritise mental and emotional well-being. Seeking peace through dhikr (remembrance of Allah), prayer, and connecting with loved ones plays a crucial role in cultivating emotional stability, which in turn supports overall health.

In conclusion, by embracing health and well-being through the Sunnah practices, we're not only nurturing our bodies but also fostering a deeper connection to our Creator. Through balanced nutrition, regular physical activity, and a consistent commitment to the teachings of Islam, we can embark on a lifelong journey of health and well-being that encompasses all dimensions of our lives.

Chapter Twelve

Conclusion

In conclusion, adopting a Sunnah-based approach to nutrition and fitness offers far more than a mere set of physical guidelines. It provides a comprehensive framework that nurtures our bodies, minds, and spirits. The teachings of the Prophet Muhammad (PBUH) encompass a holistic view of health, where the integration of physical well-being, mental clarity, and spiritual growth creates a path toward true wellness. By embracing these practices, we can attain a balanced, harmonious life that enhances our daily routines and fosters lasting physical and spiritual health.

The journey toward better health through the Sunnah is a gradual yet deeply rewarding process. It's not about following complex regimens but rather embracing simple, natural habits rooted in Islam's teachings. The prophetic practices, which include mindful eating, fasting, regular physical activity, and proper sleep hygiene, offer practical tools for improving energy levels, enhancing physical fitness, and cultivating a deeper sense of inner peace. These practices serve as timeless reminders that well-being is not confined to the physical body but extends to the mind and soul.

Mindful eating is one of the cornerstones of the Sunnah when it comes to nutrition. The Prophet Muhammad (PBUH) encouraged us to eat in moderation, to chew our food properly, and to be mindful of how and when we eat. These simple habits, such as eating in small portions and avoiding overeating, contribute to a healthier body and promote mental clarity. Eating mindfully allows our bodies to fully process the food, enabling better digestion and nutrient absorption. This contributes to both physical vitality and cognitive focus. The Sunnah teaches us to appreciate food, avoid excess, and make eating conscious, which ultimately nurtures our relationship with sustenance.

Fasting, another important Sunnah practice, offers spiritual and physical benefits. While the spiritual rewards of fasting during Ramadan are well known, the physical benefits are equally significant. Intermittent fasting, a practice that is encouraged in the Sunnah, has been shown to improve metabolic health, support weight management, and increase energy levels. Fasting allows the body to reset, promote cellular repair, and enhance overall health. Beyond these physical benefits, it fosters discipline, self-control, and a closer connection to Allah (SWT). It serves as a reminder of the importance of spiritual nourishment and the power of self-restraint.

Physical activity is another crucial aspect of the Sunnah-based approach to health. The Prophet Muhammad (PBUH) emphasised the importance of regular exercise, such as walking, horseback riding, archery, and swimming. These activities promote cardiovascular health, increase strength, and support overall fitness. Engaging in regular physical activity not only boosts our energy and stamina but also has positive effects on our mental well-being. Exercise helps reduce stress, improves mood, and enhances cognitive function, making it essential to a balanced lifestyle.

Sleep hygiene, as outlined in the Sunnah, is equally important for maintaining a healthy mind and body. The Prophet Muhammad (PBUH) taught us to establish a regular sleep routine, to sleep early and wake up early. This practice helps synchronise the body's natural rhythms and improves the quality of sleep, which in turn supports physical health and mental clarity. A good night's sleep enhances immune function, promotes emotional stability, and improves cognitive performance. The Sunnah encourages us to prioritise rest, not just as a physical need but as a way to rejuvenate our minds and souls.

As you begin to implement the principles outlined in this eBook, it's important to remember that the journey towards better health is a gradual one. You don't need to make drastic changes overnight but focus on small, intentional steps aligning with the Sunnah. Each positive habit you incorporate into your life, no matter how small, will significantly improve your overall well-being. These practices are not meant to be a burden but an opportunity to enhance your life in ways that are simple, sustainable, and spiritually rewarding.

By living in alignment with the Sunnah, you're not merely adopting a set of health practices; you're embracing a way of life that honours the teachings of Islam. You're cultivating a lifestyle that prioritises balance, mindfulness, and gratitude in every aspect of your existence. The Sunnah-based approach to health promotes a physically vibrant and spiritually fulfilling life. As you make these habits a part of your daily routine, you'll experience a transformation in your energy, well-being, and connection to your faith.

It's important to approach these practices with consistency and intention. True transformation takes time, and the key to success lies in perseverance. By embracing the principles of the Sunnah, you're not only improving your physical health but also nurturing your spiritual growth. Your journey toward better health is a reflection of your commitment to living in harmony with Allah's guidance, leading to a more fulfilling and meaningful life.

In conclusion, adopting a Sunnah-based approach to nutrition, fitness, and overall well-being offers profound benefits beyond physical health. By embracing the practices of mindful eating, fasting, regular exercise, and good sleep hygiene, we can foster balance in our lives, cultivate inner peace, and strengthen our connection to our faith. As you integrate these habits into your daily life, remember that small, consistent changes can lead to lasting improvements. By living in alignment with the Sunnah, you're taking steps toward better health and embracing a life full of purpose, balance, and spiritual growth.

Find Out More

Website: www.barakahinbusiness.com

Socials: @barakahinbusiness

If you enjoyed this book, kindly leave a review to help expand our reach so others may benefit also.

www.ingramcontent.com/pod-product-compliance
Lightning Source LLC
Chambersburg PA
CBHW070043040426
42333CB00041B/2303